Praise for *The Great Work of Your Life*

"I am moved and inspired by *The Great Work of Your Life,* the clarity and beauty of the lives lived in it, and the timeless dharma it teaches."
—**JACK KORNFIELD**, author of *A Path with Heart*

"Stephen Cope has brought the full force of his brilliant mind and expansive heart to capture the wisdom and spirit of one of history's most revered and insightful scriptures. *The Great Work of Your Life* is a remarkable testament to the power of these teachings and the timeless light they shed on how we each can craft our most glorious life. This is a must-read for anyone aspiring to lasting happiness and real fulfillment."
—**ROD STRYKER**, author of *The Four Desires*

"This book extends an impassioned, compelling promise: It is possible to live this life as a direct expression of your heart and spirit. Through masterful storytelling about extraordinary and 'ordinary' individuals, Stephen Cope unfolds perennial wisdom teachings found in the Bhagavad Gita that can illuminate your path. Not just inspiring, this book is a fascinating read!" —**TARA BRACH**, PhD, author of *Radical Acceptance*

"Stephen Cope's brilliant re-interpretation of the Bhagavad Gita for modern seekers is the next best thing to having the great god Krishna himself appear in your chariot—or the front seat of your car—and give you an inspirational pep talk as you commute to work. A master storyteller, Cope examines the lives of ordinary and extraordinary human beings through the lens of the Gita's ancient wisdom to illuminate how each of us can identify and manifest our unique calling—leaving his readers both humbled and inspired."
—**ANNE CUSHMAN**, author of *Enlightenment for Idiots: A Novel*

"Stephen Cope's genius is to connect the ancient tale of Krishna, Arjuna, and their mythic dilemmas to our very own lives through figures we not only admire but can relate to. *The Great Work Of Your Life* fearlessly bridges this gap, and its arc is incandescent."
—**CHIP HARTRANFT**, translator, *The Yoga-Sūtra of Patañjali*

"Who else could bring the ancient wisdom of the Bhagavad Gita to bear on the lives of such a diverse cast of seekers in such a captivating way? Stephen Cope is a masterful storyteller who grabbed me from the first chapter and held me until the very end. His friends became my friends, his heroes my own, and their triumphs and sorrows touched me deeply. And of course throughout, he gently reminds us all that these profound teachings can help us show up for our own dharma and lead us to do 'small things with great love.'" —**LINDA SPARROWE**, editor in chief, *Yoga International* and author of *The Woman's Book of Yoga and Health*

"*The Great Work of Your Life* is a timely and timeless must-read book. Within its pages, Stephen Cope contemplates the profound meaning of the Bhaghavad Gita, as it applies to our modern life. Exploring the call of dharma, he shows Krishna's step-by-step teaching in a way that will uplift you from within. It's essential for those new to yoga and inspiring for the seasoned practitioner and yoga teacher."

—**PATRICIA WALDEN**, international yoga teacher and co-author of *The Woman's Book of Yoga and Health*

"Stephen Cope presents an insightful look at the role of dharma as explained by Krishna to Arjuna in the timeless scripture, the Bhagavad Gita. Skillfully interweaving Arjuna's story of conflict and doubt with stories of both great and ordinary men and women, Cope illustrates how the rich wisdom of the Gita can transform our actions into spiritual practice and guide us to ultimate freedom and fulfillment."

—**PANDIT RAJMANI TIGUNAIT**, chairman and spiritual head, Himalayan Institute

"*The Great Work of Your Life* masterfully unfolds the stories of everyday people like you and me, as well as those whom we cherish as our heroes and heroines, revealing the doubts, fears, trials, and passions we will all face when we dare to live an authentic life of purpose and meaning. It will deeply inspire your heart, soul, and mind and lead you ever more deeply into finding and celebrating your own dharma."

—**RICHARD MILLER, PhD,** author of *Yoga Nidra: A Meditative Practice for Deep Relaxation and Healing,* president, Integrative Restoration Institute, and co-founder, International Association of Yoga Therapy

"This is a captivating and compassionate guide to the deepest questions of our existence. Stephen Cope ingeniously helps us to 'remember' who we really are, uncovering genuine happiness and expressing it through our dharma, our authentic work in the world."

—SARAH POWERS, author of *Insight Yoga*

"Stephen Cope hands us the secret keys of understanding and wisdom found in the sacred pages of the ancient Bhagavad Gita. He asks us the right questions, provokes, and motivates us with courage not to retreat from the world but to advance with profound enthusiasm."

—LILIAS FOLAN, PBS host and author of *Lilias! Yoga: Your Guide to Enhancing Body, Mind, and Spirit in Midlife and Beyond*

"Cope weaves together personal narratives of ordinary and extraordinary lives within the framework of the Bhagavad Gita, making the timeless scripture even more relevant to the intricacies of our twenty-first century lifestyle. A pertinent book, for NOW!"

—NISCHALA JOY DEVI, teacher, author of *The Healing Path of Yoga* and *The Secret Power of Yoga*

"*The Great Work of Your Life* is a portal into the soul of yoga. It reveals how fresh and versatile the wisdom of the Bhagavad Gita is for people of any era or stage of life. This book is a must-read for anyone wishing to penetrate the mystery of what the ancients called karma and dharma and we moderns call living an authentic life." —SCOTT BLOSSOM, LAc, CAS

THE GREAT WORK OF YOUR LIFE

BANTAM BOOKS NEW YORK

THE
GREAT
WORK
—— OF ——
YOUR
LIFE

A GUIDE FOR THE JOURNEY
TO YOUR TRUE CALLING

STEPHEN COPE

Published in the United States by Bantam Books, an imprint of
The Random House Publishing Group, a division of
Random House, Inc., New York.

BANTAM BOOKS and the rooster colophon are registered trademarks
of Random House, Inc.

Page 271 constitutes an extension of this copyright page.

Library of Congress Cataloging-in-Publication Data
Cope, Stephen.
The great work of your life : a guide for the journey to your true calling /
Stephen Cope. — 1st ed.
p.   cm.
ISBN 978-0-553-80751-6 — ISBN 978-0-345-53568-9 (ebook)
1. Spiritual biography—Hinduism.   2. Vocation—Hinduism.   3. Bhagavadgita—
Criticism, interpretation, etc.   I. Title.
BL1170.C67 2012
294.5'44—dc23
2012000863

Printed in the United States of America on acid-free paper

www.bantamdell.com

4 6 8 9 7 5

Book design by Liz Cosgrove

Dedicated to my earliest mentors,

Wilson Martindale Compton

and Helen Harrington Compton,

who demonstrated in their lives the nobility of work

Every man has a vocation to be someone:

but he must understand clearly that in order to fulfill this

vocation he can only be one person: himself.

—Thomas Merton

—— CONTENTS ——

PART IV

The Third Pillar: "Let Go of the Fruits" 125

PART V

The Fourth Pillar: "Turn It Over to God" 201

This is a book about dharma—about vocations and callings. It contains many stories of illustrious lives—true stories of lives that many of us already know and admire. It also contains stories of what I have called "ordinary lives"—lives that are in many ways just like yours and mine. I have included so-called ordinary lives for a reason: It is impossible to understand the living truth of dharma without getting close to the lives and experiences of real practitioners. But in writing an "experience-near" account of these ordinary lives, I have had to face a difficult challenge: how to tell the stories of my friends, students, and colleagues without invading their privacy. I have chosen in almost every case in this book to create composite characters—sticking as closely as I can to the emotional and psychological truth of real experience, while creating essentially fictional characters and dialogues. Many of us will see aspects of ourselves in these characters and conversations, of course, but, aside from a handful (whom I have given their real names), the "ordinary" characters in this book do not, and are not meant to, represent any actual persons.

One additional proviso: The book that you are about to read is an examination of dharma in the light of the teachings of the two-thousand-year-old Bhagavad Gita. But this book in no way purports to be a scholarly or technical exegesis of the Gita. Many fine scholarly treatments of this scripture are readily available. This book is something altogether

different. What follows is an experience-near account of one practitioner's thirty-year engagement with the Gita. Its purpose is simple: to
awaken the mainstream reader to the genius of this magnificent text,
and to elucidate—through stories—some of its most important principles for living. It is my hope that the reader, once alerted to its genius,
will go on to investigate the Gita's complex and subtle teachings more
closely—and at that point, more scholarly treatments of the text will
become useful and, indeed, invaluable.

What do you fear most in this life?

What is your biggest fear? Right now.

When I pose that question to myself, the answer is this. I'm afraid that I'll die without having lived fully. OK, I'm also afraid of pain—and of dying a difficult death. But that's for later. Mostly, right now, I'm afraid that I may be missing some magnificent possibility. That perhaps I have not risked enough to find it. That maybe I've lived too safe a life.

Thomas Merton says, "What you fear is an indication of what you seek."

In my case I think this is certainly true. And deep in middle age, I can feel the *seeker* in me become just ever-so-slightly desperate.

One of the ways this desperation shows up is in my reading. I've always been a reader, to be sure, but lately the temperature on the dial has been inched up. Something new: I've become a *voracious* reader. I am hungry to hear other people's answers to my questions—particularly other people who might be experts in this problem of possibilities: Thomas Merton, Garry Wills, Henry David Thoreau, Annie Dillard, Jean-Pierre de Caussade, Karen Armstrong, Emily Dickinson, Robert Frost. These are just a few exemplars of the struggle to live fully who tumble around in my head. What can they teach me about desperation and fulfillment?

And so, I read. Usually from about 8:00 to 11:00 every night—often propped up in bed, with an unruly stack of books perched on the table next to me. I read with pen in hand, and have lively conversations with my authors. I scribble in margins; I make exclamation points and stars; I draw arrows from one page to another, tracking arguments.

Every now and then, in my quest for answers, I stumble across a sentence that stands up and shouts at me from the page. Here is a sentence I read recently in the pages of the Gnostic Gospel of Thomas.

"If you bring forth what is within you, what you bring forth will save you; if you do not bring forth what is within you, what you do not bring forth will destroy you."

What?

I sat up in bed. I circled the whole sentence.

If you bring forth what is within you, it will save you; if you do not bring forth what is within you, it will destroy you.

I have to admit that the second phrase of the sentence hit me the hardest. It will destroy me?

In retrospect, I realize that I felt the punch of that second phrase only because I had genuinely experienced moments of the first.

I *do* know the experience of bringing forth what is within me. For most of my life, these bringing-forth moments have been fleeting. But twice I've had the experience sustained over a period of years. Both times this happened while I was writing a book. Writing required everything I had, and then some. It flayed me alive. But I kept coming back again and again. I kept bringing forth the best that was in me. I can't say whether the books that came forth are good or not. Some say yes and some say no. It doesn't matter. It seems that it was the *effort required to bring them forth* itself that saved me. I noticed later that *having written them* did not really bring me squat, even though most people—including myself—thought that it should.

I have friends who are right now bringing forth what is within them. Anyone can see it in their faces. These are people who leap out of bed in the morning. They are digging down. Connecting with their own particular genius, and bringing it into the world. They are bringing forth their point of view, their idiosyncratic wisdom. They are living out their vocations. And let me tell you, they are *lit up*.

This way of lit-up living can happen in any sphere. Not a single one of my lit-up friends is writing a book, by the way. One of my friends, Mark, is busy building a new institution—an alternative prep school. My friend Sandy is mastering the art of nursing hospice patients. (Can you imagine leaping out of bed in the morning to confront the dying? She does. And actually, I *can* imagine it.) One of my friends is busy mastering Beethoven's string quartets. Day and night she practices. My friend David is on fire—creating an entirely new genre of landscape painting. Alan is mastering the art of gardening and just, really, the art of living life as a naturalist. My sister Arlie is mastering the to-me-incomprehensible task of parenting an adolescent—but with such relish you cannot believe it.

Have you had periods in life when you leapt out of bed in the morning to embrace your day? Once this happens to you, once you live this way, even for a few hours, you will never really be satisfied with any other way of living. Everything else will seem vaguely wan and gray. Everything else will seem, as Henry David Thoreau said, like "a distraction."

Maybe you're saying to yourself: It's not that black-and-white. You can't live this way all the time. Maybe this guy (me) is just in a dry period—something like what the Christian saints called "a desert experience." Maybe these dry periods are just as productive, really—and every bit as necessary—as the wet periods. Maybe you can't even dream of bringing forth what is within you without a requisite amount of aridity.

This is a good point. Besides, it is impossible to tell from the outside who *is* and who *is not* "bringing forth what is within them." And, in truth, leaping out of bed in the morning really has very little to do with it.

But still. There is a vast difference between the desert experience of the saints and watching endless reruns on TV, isn't there?

But for now, here's an experiment. Stop reading for a minute, and ask yourself these questions: Am I living fully right now? Am I bringing forth everything I *can* bring forth? Am I digging down into that ineffable inner treasure-house that I know is in there? That trove of genius? Am I living my life's calling? Am I willing to go to any lengths to offer my genius to the world?

For me, truthfully, when I pose these questions to myself, I hear my-self say (as I shuffle from one foot to the other), "Well, yes, I'm just in the process of instituting a new *plan* that will bring me fully alive again." Hmm. That's a no, isn't it? But *why* is it a no for me just now? And what can I do about it? Do I have any control over these things? Is it just, well, karma?

I see my own concerns about fulfillment played out nearly every day of my professional life. I work at one of the largest holistic retreat centers in America—the Kripalu Center for Yoga and Health. We see more than 35,000 people a year here in our sprawling, former-Jesuit monastery perched high up in the Berkshire Hills of Western Massachusetts. Our guests come for various kinds of retreats: yoga, meditation, self-inquiry, couples' work, healthy living. And almost every single one of them comes here in some phase of the mission to find this secret, hidden, inner possibility spoken of in the Gospel of Thomas.

A true story: Whenever I teach our program participants here at Kripalu, I begin by asking them to name what they've come for. Seventy-five percent say it straight out: "I want to come home to my true self." Over and over again in almost those exact words. "To come home to my true self." Where have these people been? The same place I've been, lately, I guess: Unclear. Confused. Paralyzed by doubt. Gliding. Drifting. Mesmerized by the old tried-and-true distractions. (And maybe some of us have truly been in the desert.)

Most of our guests come to a yoga retreat because they know by now that the yoga tradition is almost entirely concerned—obsessed, really—with the problem of living a fulfilled life. The yoga tradition is a virtual catalog of the various methods human beings have discovered over the past 3,000 years to function on all cylinders. This includes everything from the world's weirdest diets to the most sublime forms of prayer and meditation—and ecstatic experience. One of the greatest archetypes of the yoga tradition is the *jivan mukta*—the soul awake in this lifetime. *The soul awake.* I like this aspect of yoga, because it means awake *in this lifetime*—not in some afterlife, or heavenly realm, or exalted mental state. And so these contemporary seekers come to yoga, seeking—as I did, and do—inspiration for living.

The yoga tradition is very, very interested in the idea of an inner possibility harbored within every human soul. Yogis insist that every single human being has a unique vocation. They call this *dharma*. Dharma is a potent Sanskrit word that is packed tight with meaning, like one of those little sponge animals that expands to six times its original size when you add water. Dharma means, variously, "path," "teaching," or "law." For our purposes in this book it will mean primarily "vocation," or "sacred duty." It means, most of all—and in all cases—*truth*. Yogis believe that our greatest responsibility in life is to this inner possibility—this dharma— and they believe that every human being's duty is to utterly, fully, and completely embody his own idiosyncratic dharma.

Most of the people I teach here at Kripalu catch on to the idea of dharma right away. They often say that they feel comforted that someone has taken the trouble to give a name to this urgent and irksome call that has flashed in and out of their brain for so long, like a lamp with a bad connection.

Not only did yogis *name* this hidden inner genius, but they created a detailed method for fulfilling it. In fact, the ancient treatise in which this method is spelled out is hands down the most important and well-loved scripture in the world of yoga.

I am referring, of course, to the 2,000-year-old treatise on yoga called the Bhagavad Gita, or Song of God. It is the world's greatest scripture on dharma.

In India, every villager knows the story of the Gita. It is the story of the warrior Arjuna and his divine mentor, Krishna. Arjuna is supposedly the greatest warrior of his time, but really, he is just astonishingly like we are: neurotic as hell, and full of every doubt and fear you can imagine. The Gita tells how Krishna taught Arjuna—*even* Arjuna—to embrace his sacred vocation. In India, Krishna and Arjuna are pictured everywhere and their story is played out in temple carvings and icons of every variety, so even illiterate folk know the tale. For two thousand years, people have read or chanted the Gita daily, just as we read our Bible, or Torah, or Koran. The Gita is the one book Gandhi took with him to prison, and one of the few that Henry David Thoreau took to Walden Pond.

The first time I heard the story of Krishna and Arjuna was in a World Lit course in college. I read the book. I listened to all the lectures. And I probably even did well in the class. But quite honestly I never got what all the fuss was about. All that has changed. Deep in middle age, I *get* it. Reading a book like this is as important to me as breathing oxygen.

The Bhagavad Gita expounds an unequaled method for bringing forth dharma. At the beginning of the story, Arjuna is paralyzed by doubt. Like Hamlet, he cannot act. Arjuna has tried to live a good life up to this point—has tried to live out his warrior-dharma as best he can. But at the beginning of our story, the world has momentarily crushed him. Luckily for Arjuna, Krishna is at his side at the very moment of that crunch. The handsome Krishna is disguised as a charioteer, and he becomes Arjuna's spiritual teacher, his psychoanalyst, his coach, his goad, his mentor. But we—the reader—know that Krishna is actually none other than God.

As the tale opens, our friend Arjuna has collapsed onto the floor of his chariot. Arjuna is undone by the doubts and conflicts he faces about his own actions—his own calling—on the field of a great battle that is about to be engaged. "What am I really called to *do* in this circumstance?" he asks Krishna. "Do I fight this battle, or not?" How do I act in such a way that I do not destroy my own soul and the soul of the world? How do I act in such a way that I fulfill my dharma?

The Bhagavad Gita is a brilliant teaching on the problems of *doing*. There is so much talk these days about *being*. (And for good reason.) But what a treat to discover a great scripture about *doing*. "All that is worthwhile," says the great Jesuit scholar and paleontologist Teilhard de Chardin, "is action." In fact, there is no being in this world without doing. Let's get real: Most of our lives are spent in doing. From the point of view of the Gita, the most sublime kind of doing is really a perfect expression of authentic being. Does this sound a little abstract? It will become very concrete as we sort through the argument of the Gita.

Arjuna has many excellent questions for Krishna—questions to which we, too, would like answers: Who am I, for God's sake? And how can I authentically express all that I truly am?

Over the course of eighteen enchanting chapters, Krishna and Arjuna sort through these questions. Krishna gives some awesome talks about action versus inaction, about doubt and faith, about knowledge and love. Arjuna hedges his way from chapter to chapter, until about halfway through the book, when Krishna at last has to really get stern with him. In the famous Chapter Eleven, Krishna pulls out his big guns—and one of the world's most stunning theophanies explodes into the consciousness of a bewildered Arjuna. Now Arjuna really understands who he is messing with. From here on out tumble some of the world's most inspiring teachings about devotion, love, work, and duty.

By the end of the book, these two friends have sorted out the Truth. We readers feel sorted out, too.

If you look around, you might notice that suddenly you're seeing the Bhagavad Gita everywhere. Everyone still reads it in World Lit courses, naturally. But more than that. I've heard that it is rapidly replacing *The Art of War* on the bookshelves of corporate executives.

I hope this is true. It indicates that we're finally beginning to bring spiritual practice into the center of our everyday lives—moving away from the misapprehension that spiritual life only happens in church, or on the meditation cushion, or on retreat. Or that full-time spiritual pursuits are strictly the province of those living a so-called religious life. No. Arjuna is the archetype of the spiritual man *in action.*

In fact, the Bhagavad Gita was written precisely to show us how to make the world of action (the marketplace, the workplace, the family) an arena for spiritual development. Indeed, it portrays the "battlefield" of life—real life, everyday life—as the most potent venue for transformation.

Reading the Gita brings into stark relief a misapprehension we have about our everyday lives—a mistaken belief about the nature of fulfillment itself. Our fantasies about fulfillment often center around dreams of wealth, power, fame, and leisure. In these fantasies, a fulfilling life is one in which we acquire so much freedom and leisure that we no longer have to work and strive. Finally, once we've worked most of our lives to extricate ourselves from the demands of ordinary life, we can relax by our own personally monogrammed swimming pool—with the gates of our country-club community firmly locked behind us—and there, at last, find true happiness, and real fulfillment, perhaps contemplating the clear blue sky.

The teachings of the Gita point to a much more interesting truth: People actually feel happiest and most fulfilled when meeting the challenge of their dharma *in the world,* when bringing highly concentrated effort to some compelling activity for which they have a true calling. For most of us this means our work in the world. And by work, of course, I do not mean only "job." For many of us—as for Arjuna—the challenges of our vocation in the world require the development of a profound degree of mastery. Those who have had a taste of this kind of mastery have experienced moments when effort becomes effortless: joyful, gifted, and unbounded. These moments of effortless effort are so sublime that they draw us even more deeply into the possibilities of our vocations. At the end of life, most of us will find that we have felt most filled up by the challenges and successful struggles for mastery, creativity, and full expression of our dharma in the world. Fulfillment happens not in *retreat* from the world, but in *advance*—and profound engagement.

The two-thousand-year-old Bhagavad Gita brings us a series of surprising principles for living an optimal life, and for transforming skillful action into spiritual practice.

In 2005, I became director of a new institute at Kripalu, called The Institute for Extraordinary Living. Our goal was to do rigorous scientific research on fulfillment—to understand skillful living of the Gita brand and to examine the ways in which it may show up in our time. Are there some people who really *do* live their dharma authentically, and in a fulfilling fashion? Do we know them? Are there any characteristics that consistently mark their lives? Do these people, in fact, jump out of bed in the morning? What might Krishna and Arjuna's teachings on dharma mean for us?

Our quest to understand these things has led me to an intensive study of so-called "great lives"—the lives of those who have obviously brought forth their genius into the world. You've heard briefly from a few of these characters already in this introduction—Thoreau, de Chardin, Merton—and you'll hear much more from them and many other such "greats" throughout the course of this book. I have learned a tremendous amount from my study of these well-known exemplars of dharma, including the very reassuring fact that the whole lot of them had just as many doubts and neuroses and fears as the rest of us. Often more.

Along the way, I have looked, too, at what we might call "ordinary lives." You and me. And what a bonfire of inspiration came from this study of ordinary lives. It turns out that among so-called *ordinary* lives, there are many, many *great* ones. Indeed, for me there is no longer really any distinction at all between great lives and ordinary lives.

I must admit that this surprised me at first. If it surprises you as well, I suggest that you look carefully about your own neighborhood. There are people all around you right now living out their vocations—strange vocations you never even imagined. It is not so easy to tell from the outside whether someone is fully engaged in his dharma. This is because dharma draws forth an ardency so deep—and sometimes so secret— that it often cannot be detected by ordinary eyes. Perhaps the neighbor who you think is profoundly strange because he stays inside and collects stamps and sometimes forgets to put out his garbage and doesn't come to the annual block party—perhaps he is utterly involved in his sacred calling. Perhaps his single-minded efforts have lifted stamp collecting to an entirely new level of genius. Perhaps he has penetrated the mystery of stamps, or is about to do so. Inside he glows, but you cannot see it. But I tell you this: You are more likely to have X-ray eyes for such things if you are also pursuing your own dharma with the same ardency.

And this brings us to you: Do you fear that you may have missed the boat? That you've become unmoored from your true calling and are drifting aimlessly out to sea?

Here is another surprise that may buoy you up. Most of the ordinary people whom I have studied, when first confronted with the notion of dharma, imagined that for them to claim their dharma probably meant inventing an entirely new life. Giving up their job selling insurance and moving to Paris to paint. Quitting their job as a hospice nurse and sailing around the world solo. Not so. As it turns out, most people are already living very close to their dharma. Really. Within spitting range. What is the problem, then? These same people, close as they are to the deepest mystery of dharma, know very little about it. They don't name it. They don't own it. They don't live it intentionally. Their own sacred calling is hiding in plain sight. They keep just missing it. And, as we will see, when it comes to dharma, missing by an inch is as good as missing by a mile. Aim is everything.

Come with me, then, and with my fellow students of fulfillment as we tell the story of Krishna and Arjuna, and as we tell stories of great lives that vividly reflect the principles of living as they are laid out in the Bhagavad Gita. Bring your fears and neuroses and doubts; do not leave that excellent fodder behind. Bring your desperation and your most ardent wishes for a full life. Gather 'round the fire with the rest of us ordinary human beings, as we investigate the not-so-far-fetched possibility of becoming fully alive.

PART I

Krishna's Counsel
on the Field of Battle

As the curtain rises on Chapter One of the Bhagavad Gita, we are at the scene of an impending battle—the fabled battle of Kurukshetra, in the North Indian Kingdom of Kuru. Krishna, the charioteer, and Arjuna, the young warrior, have driven their chariot to the edge of the battleground. Arjuna surveys the scene, and speaks urgently to his charioteer: "I see omens of chaos, Krishna." As we survey the battlefield in our mind's eye, we feel—with Arjuna—a visceral sense of foreboding. The narrator has already told us that the forces of light and the forces of darkness are about to collide, and that this battle will tear the fabric of the world.

As early readers of the Gita would have been all too aware, this is indeed no ordinary battle. The battle of Kurukshetra is the definitive struggle of its age. It marks the end of one great mythic era (*yuga*, or world age) and the beginning of another. The battle of Kurukshetra ushers in the Dark Age—the *Kali-yuga*—the last of the four great eras foreseen by the Seers of ancient India.

Imagine our two heroes as they prepare for this world-shattering conflict.

Krishna, the charioteer, is dark-skinned and handsome. He is steady. Regal. Unwavering. We'll find out later, of course, that he is God in one of his many disguises.

Arjuna, our bold warrior, too, is handsome. But not so steady as

Krishna. He is young and brash and immature. He is highly prized by his family, and idealized by the common people. He is something of a golden boy. (Do you have one of these in your family? They can be terribly irritating.) There is no doubt, from the very outset, that Arjuna is an exceptionally brave warrior, though he does not yet possess the supernormal powers of the yogi. All that is yet to come.

"Krishna," says Arjuna as the narrative opens, "halt my chariot between the armies! Far enough for me to see these men who lust for war . . ."

Arjuna surveys the scene of the impending battle. And what does he see? A sight that undoes him. Arjuna sees his own kinsmen arrayed against him. He sees, as he says to Krishna, "fathers, grandfathers, teachers, uncles, brothers, sons, grandsons, and friends" gathered in the opposing army.

His own family has taken up arms against him? How did we get to this disastrous crossroads?

We need a little background here. The Kingdom of Kuru has been ripped apart by a now-generations-old conflict between two different but closely related lines of the royal family: the Pandavas and the Kauravas. The Pandavas, as you have probably guessed, are Arjuna's family, and they have come to be known as "the forces of light." The Kauravas—their conniving cousins—have by this point earned their name as "the forces of darkness." They have illegally usurped the throne of Kuru, and destroyed the peace and well-being of the people.

As Arjuna surveys the impending conflict between the Pandavas and the Kauravas, he sees "omens of chaos." He sees the breakdown of the harmony and order of family and kingdom—an order highly prized for the peace and well-being that it fosters. He sees, too, his own family deeply stained by the forces of disorder—by avarice, and the lust for power, land, and fortune. The forces of greed, hatred, and delusion are the destroyers of the world order and purveyors of suffering.

Arjuna, observing all of this, is loath to become part of the pernicious disorder infecting the kingdom. He is reluctant to take his part in this battle, even though it is manifestly his sacred duty.

"Conflicting sacred duties confound my reason!" Arjuna cries to Krishna.

A cry of doubt! Arjuna is split down the middle. How should he act?

As a great warrior, Arjuna has always known that his sacred duty is to fight on the side of "right" in a just war. And according to the rules of war so clearly laid out in the scriptures—rules that are as close to Arjuna as his own heart—this is, indeed, a just war. The peace of the kingdom has been profoundly disrupted by the unjust usurpation of the throne. The forces of greed and disorder have triumphed. The people of the realm will suffer as a result of this unjust usurpation. It is Arjuna's duty to fight.

And yet. He is confronted with a problem above and beyond the ordinary challenges of war. He sees that his own people are standing against him. Will he kill them? If he does, he will have committed the heinous sin of fratricide, and he will take on the karma of this act, and suffer for many lifetimes to come.

However, if he does *not* act, he will betray his "code"—the sacred duty that has given his very life meaning.

Arjuna is caught on the horns of a vicious dilemma. "We don't know which weight is worse to bear," Arjuna says to Krishna, "our conquering them or their conquering us."

Arjuna feels the conflict viscerally. "Krishna," he says:

"My limbs sink,
My mouth is parched,
My body trembles,
The hair bristles on my flesh.
The magic bow slips
From my hand, my skin burns,
I cannot stand still,
My mind reels."

Arjuna sees clearly that having executed his sacred duty, having slain his own kinsmen, he will not himself be able to go on living: "We will not want to live if we kill the sons of Dhritarashtra assembled before us."

What should he do?

Arjuna does, perhaps, the most sensible thing possible: He falls to the floor of his chariot.

"I cannot fight this fight," he cries to Krishna.

And then Arjuna falls silent.

ONE

The Four Pillars of Dharma

From the very beginning of the Bhagavad Gita we can see that it is going to be a teaching about dharma—about sacred duty. Anybody can see that the first chapter is a device used by the author to set up the problem of vocation. How do we know, finally, to what actions we are called in this life? The author knows that we'll identify with Arjuna's dilemma: How do we choose between two difficult courses of action? What are the consequences of an inability to choose, or of choosing poorly? Who can effectively guide us in making these choices? Finally, in any ultimate sense, does it really matter what choices we make with our life?

At the outset of this tale, the narrator describes Arjuna as paralyzed by doubt. He has come to a crossroads in his life, and is forced to choose between two difficult paths. And for the time being Arjuna has demurred. He is stuck on the floor of the chariot, unable to act at all. From the beginning, then, it is clear that the narrator sees Arjuna's central affliction as the problem of doubt.

For those of us who study the contemplative traditions, this is exciting. Something new! Until the writing of the Bhagavad Gita, the Eastern contemplative traditions—both yoga and Buddhism—had almost universally seen *grasping* as the central affliction or "torment" in the lives of human beings. These traditions had come to really understand the afflictive nature of desire, craving, grasping, greed, lust.

Grasping will come into Krishna's teaching, to be sure. But at the outset of the tale, Arjuna's central torment is not grasping. Or even its flip side—fear and aversion. No, it's clear to us that Arjuna is not really so much *afraid* as he is *immobilized* in a web of doubt. Stuck on the floor of the chariot.

In the fourth chapter, Krishna will state the principle clearly: "Doubt afflicts the person who lacks faith and can ultimately destroy him."

This doubt of which Krishna speaks is the outward and visible sign of an inner struggle. And if this inner struggle is not resolved, it will (as St. Thomas declares in his Gospel) destroy him.

The stakes are serious. It will be important for us to understand the exact nature of this doubt that afflicts our hero.

Notice that "doubt," as used in the Gita, is somewhat different than our ordinary Western understanding of doubt. When we think of doubt, we most often think of what we might better call "healthy skepticism"—a lively mind, closely investigating all options. That is not quite what the Gita means. Doubt, as understood here, really means "stuck"—not skeptical. Doubt in this tradition is sometimes defined as "a thought that *touches both sides of a dilemma at the same time.*" In yogic analysis, doubt is often called "the paralyzing affliction." Paralysis is, indeed, its chief characteristic. It follows, then, that doubt is the central affliction of all men and women of action.

The Catholic Encyclopedia weighs in convincingly on this issue. Apparently, doubt is an issue for Catholics as well as Hindus: "Doubt," it reads, "[is a] state in which the mind is suspended between two contradictory propositions and unable to assent to either of them."

Catholics and yogis are apparently in agreement about this phenomenon of doubt.

The Catholic Encyclopedia continues at great length. "Doubt," it says, "is opposed to certitude, or the adhesion of the mind to a proposition without misgiving as to its truth."

Here the Catholics make an opposition of doubt and certitude. This, I think, is very helpful.

And listen to the definition of certitude that follows. Certitude: "the adhesion of the mind to a proposition without misgiving as to its truth."

Without misgiving!

In Arjuna we have a hero whose doubt is writ large. He is split down the middle. And it will take the entire eighteen chapters of the Bhagavad Gita before he gets to certitude. But what a thrill when he does.

"Krishna," says Arjuna at the very end of the Gita, "my delusion is destroyed, and by your grace I have regained memory; I stand here, my doubt dispelled, ready to act on your words!"

My doubt dispelled!

Until I began to wrestle with the teachings of the Bhagavad Gita, I thought that doubt was the least of my problems. Grasping and aversion, the classic afflictions pointed to by the earlier yoga tradition, were much more obvious in my life. However, as I have begun to investigate the Gita's view of doubt, and as I begin to understand what doubt really is, I see it at work everywhere. I've begun to see the ways—both small and large—in which I am paralyzed from action on a daily basis. Split. Replete with misgivings. Unsure. A foot on both sides of various dilemmas.

We can see why the yoga tradition has called doubt "the invisible affliction." It is slippery. Hidden. Sneaky. Indeed, it is this very hidden quality that gives doubt its power. I know people who have been stuck in doubt their entire lifetime. Each of these unfortunate individuals—some of them my very own friends and family—came at some point to a crossroads. They came to this crossroads and found themselves rooted there, with one foot firmly planted on each side of the intersection. Alas, they never moved off the dime. They procrastinated. Dithered. Finally, they put a folding chair smack in the center of that crossroads and lived there for the rest of their lives. After a while, they forgot entirely that there even was a crossroads—forgot that there was a choice.

We do not suspect the ways in which doubt keeps us paralyzed. Plastered to the bottom of our various chariots. Unable to assent.

I see it all the time in the people I work with at Kripalu.

Just to give you a taste of how these things show up, let me give you a thumbnail sketch of one of these people, a woman whom I will call Katherine. She has recently come to one of these fateful crossroads, and has already put down her folding chair.

—— 2 ——

Katherine has been for many years the dean of a small private girls' school—a school that one of my friends calls Crunchy Granola Hall. Katherine is loved by several generations of students: mothers and daughters. For years she has lived squarely in the center of her dharma, her sacred duty. She has changed lives. Anyone who knows her would declare that she has thrived in the role of dean of this school: counseling and befriending faculty and students; helping chart the course of the school; raising money for new buildings. Now, however, she is tired. She is irritable and pissy with her faculty. She forgets to attend important meetings. She is, if truth be told, finished. In her heart of hearts she knows it. In private she admits it to me: She no longer even cares.

But Katherine is terrified. And completely unsure of what might come next. She is afraid that if she leaves the deanship, she will be devastatingly lonely. That only her cats will need her. She knows there is a new dharma calling her, and in fleeting moments she sees it out of the corner of her eye. She occasionally gets a whiff of a calling that feels more real than rain: Perhaps she could teach English literature to her young charges. She could be free of the wearying burdens of deanship. She could work only a few hours a week. She could garden (her passion)!

Katherine can occasionally visualize how perfect this would be, and how well it would meet her energies at this stage of life. English literature has been one of her most enduring loves. She could transmit it to the girls in small doses. When she visualizes this new dharma, she feels the possibility of living once again. But then the fear comes. Maybe she won't get invited to all the important powwows about the future of the school. Maybe they'll think of her as washed-up—consigned to the oblivion of the educational North Forty. And then she thinks, "Perhaps I should stick it out for another year. There will be just a little more in my retirement package, too." Katherine has been paralyzed by this conflict for more than three years, and she is not a happy woman. "Living a lie," she has even said to me after several glasses of wine.

Katherine is stuck. She might well say with Arjuna, "Conflicting sacred duties confound my reason!"

— 3 —

There are many ways to be quietly paralyzed by doubt. We might call Katherine's version Fear of Closing the Door. I see this version quite frequently. Someone has had a profound taste of living their dharma, maybe even for decades. But now that particular dharma is used up—lived out. You can smell it. This person knows that a certain dharma moment is over but has only the vaguest sense of what must be next. It increasingly begins to dawn on her that in order to find that next expression of dharma she is going to have to take a leap of some kind. She knows that she is going to have to close a door behind her before she will find the next door to open. And gradually she comes to the edge of a cliff, where she knows a leap of faith will be required. This is where she sets down in her folding chair. Will she ever get up?

Fear of Closing the Door is one version of dharma paralysis. But there are many others—countless others, really. Let me recount just a couple of these to you, so that you can get a flavor of the possibilities.

— 4 —

Katherine's story is rather dramatic. But here is a different kind of dharma problem that is perhaps closer to home for most of us. Let's call this one Denial of Dharma.

My friend Ellen and I were talking one day over brunch. I was telling her about the work of our Institute, and asking her about her own life—her own vocation. "Well, I don't really have a calling," said Ellen a little wistfully. "I wish I did. But I don't." Ellen was at that time a head nurse in the psychiatric unit of a local VA hospital. I knew—because several of her colleagues had told me—that she was greatly respected, and even loved, in the hospital. She was knowledgeable, professional, masterful. Always learning more. A hard worker. As she described herself, though, she was "just a regular old worker bee—not one of those people with a high calling."

Ellen loves to help. To support people. To love people. To be of service. Not only at work, but all around her community in Albany. She helps Jessica, our mutual friend with Alzheimer's. She takes care of Bill, her friend with a brain tumor. She keeps a watchful eye out for her adult son, Jim, and his girlfriend—helping where she can, and unobtrusively. I mean, really. Ellen is an angel for many. Her Thanksgiving table, a meal which I attend every year, is an outpouring of generosity. Ellen gets a tremendous amount of satisfaction out of lending a hand. She does it quietly, with no fanfare, and often with great humor. Her best friend, Dee, told me recently that in the early years of their friendship, she watched Ellen very closely, looking for the crack in her spirit of giving. She can't really be *that* generous, can she? She can't really enjoy giving that much. She must secretly resent it, don't you think? Finally, Dee concluded with astonishment that she actually *does* enjoy giving that much.

Now, Ellen has a brother named Henry, who is also a good friend of mine. Henry is a well-known film producer. He lives a crazily dramatic life. He is wildly and publicly successful. He is rich. He is Ellen's younger brother. But Ellen has always felt overshadowed by him. Who wouldn't?

Ellen lives with the sense that she does not have a calling, simply because her calling is not dramatic—like Henry's. But she most certainly *does* have a calling. It's clear to everyone around her. Her dharma work is everywhere. It saturates her life. She lives so much in the center of her calling that she doesn't see it. For Ellen, her *life* is her dharma. It is not just about her job, or even her career, though in her case, that career, too, is part of her dharma. Ellen is squarely in the middle of her dharma. But she has not named it, and therefore is not, in a strange sense, *doing it on purpose.* All that is left is for her to embrace her dharma. To name it. To claim it. To own it.

This is Denial of Dharma, and I see it all the time. It is a sly version of doubt. With Denial of Dharma, there is often a vagueness, a lack of clarity—and confusion about the nature of dharma itself. Ellen's boat is not really sailing trimmed to the wind. But it could be. If she just took a small step toward embracing her dharma. What stands in her way? We will examine this interesting question in some depth as we go along.

— 5 —

And finally, here is one last example of the many forms of doubt. This one we will call The Problem of Aim.

Let me introduce you to a man I will call Brian—Father Brian—who is a priest in a local Roman Catholic parish. Brian was young—as most are—when he went to seminary in Boston and committed to the priesthood. He knew he had a vocation. He felt it stirring early in his high school days, when he admired the priests at the prestigious private high school he attended. And he had always loved to be in church. The Church, as he once told me, always "had the magic" for him.

So what is the problem? Well, Brian is now forty-three years old, and he knows more about who he really is. He now says he was perhaps slightly confused about his vocation. Yes, he does love the Church, and he does believe in the Church as an important institution. But he realizes now that what he really loves, what really gets him up in the morning, is the *music* of the Church. He's an accomplished organist. Has a beautiful Irish tenor voice. He realizes now, as he leads Sunday Mass, that he would much rather be in the choir, or directing the choir, or playing the organ, than be behind the altar. "I just don't feel like a priest," he says. "I feel like a musician. I feel like a transgendered person before the operation. I look like a priest. But under the cassock, it's not quite me." He looks down from the throne where he sits as rector, and longs to be just a part of the choir.

Oops. Brian almost made it squarely to the center of his vocation. But not quite. Close—but no cigar. Brian lives in close proximity to his dharma—to his passion. But not in the passionate center of it. It has taken him quite a few years to realize this.

This is not a simple problem. In fact, Brian is actually very good at being a priest. He is a wonderful preacher—an incisive theological thinker. And though it's true that he's not gifted as a counselor, and that in obvious ways he is not interested in being a pastor, he has so many of the gifts one needs that he "passes" very well as a competent rector.

This is a problem of aim. How important is it that we live squarely in the center of our dharma? How many of us get it almost right, but not quite right? And is a miss by an inch *really* as good as a miss by a mile?

Brian has done pretty well with his dilemma, at least until recently. It seems that the older he gets, the more he longs to live squarely in the center of his dharma, and the more he feels the accumulated weight of a kind of creeping self-betrayal. In the past two years, he tells me, he has begun to feel moments of desperation about it. He is angry with God. He has periods of loss of faith. He gets depressed. And he is currently seeing a Church counselor. It is all pouring out.

Brian has finally realized that he does have the gift of a passion, *but he has not been pursuing it.* He has been trying to transcend this conflict through prayer and confession, and through being as close as possible to what he loves: sacred music. This has been, for him, like falling in love with someone who is married to someone else, and deciding that it might be enough in this lifetime just to live *next door* to the beloved.

Do you recognize Brian's problem of aim? It's a curious thing about dharma. It's almost all about aim. It appears that we will not hit the target of dharma unless we are *aiming* at it. And does hitting the target matter? It does to Brian. He is on the floor of his chariot as we speak.

Katherine, Ellen, Brian. Each one of them is stuck on the bottom of their chariots. Unable to fully assent. Lacking certitude. Their lives are colored by doubt.

There are, of course, a thousand ways of being stuck. Of being split. Freud believed that that "split" is the very nature of neurosis. And that none of us can avoid it. It is, apparently, a part of the human experience.

But is a life of certitude really possible? Krishna teaches that it is. But the key to living a life true to dharma is a complete understanding of and respect for doubt. Indeed, the only way to get to certitude is to look more and more deeply into our doubt—to shine a light into the dark corners of our self-division.

—— 6 ——

Let's revisit our friends Krishna and Arjuna. Arjuna, you will recall, is still sitting on the floor of his brightly painted chariot, his knees tucked up tight to his chest, and his arms wrapped around his legs. His head is slumped forward. Krisha stands next to him—silently—and Arjuna can feel Krishna's powerful gaze. The flags on the back of the chariot flap softly in the wind. The field of Kurukshetra—the field of battle—seems preternaturally quiet.

At the outset of our tale, Krishna has given Arjuna a sublime speech about our True Nature. But Arjuna is not in the mood for philosophy.

He has more pressing problems on his mind. He is still stuck—facing a devastating battle, and perhaps his own death. He is struggling with a seemingly impossible decision about all of it. He lives in a world of immediate difficult choices.

In desperation, Arjuna has chosen the path of *inaction*. He has put down his folding chair in the middle of the intersection. "If I can't figure out how to act, I'll do nothing at all," he has said to Krishna. But he does not feel good about this decision. This is familiar territory for most of us.

Krishna immediately points out the problem with this "do-nothing" strategy. This apparent path of *inaction* is full of *action*. Says Krishna, "No one exists for even an instant without performing action." Arjuna's inaction—our inaction—on the floor of the chariot, the center of the intersection, is action motivated by confusion, paralysis, disorder. It is full of action *and the consequences of action.*

Arjuna does not want to hear this. He turns away from Krishna, takes a deep breath, and lets out a sigh. He stretches out his legs, and then slowly hauls himself to the side of the chariot, where he dismounts. He dusts himself off, and walks around the chariot to once again survey the field of the coming battle.

Finally, Arjuna walks back to the large wooden vehicle, and sits down on the driver's intricately adorned bench, motioning to Krishna to join him there.

"OK," he says, with resignation. "So I cannot *not* act. I guess I see that. But then how do I act? How do I know *how* to act? What is the right thing to do?"

Krishna sits down next to his young charge. He is quiet for a while. Finally, he speaks.

"Arjuna," he begins his wonderful opening speech, "look to your dharma."

And with this, Krishna launches into the first of many speeches about the most revolutionary teaching of the Bhagavad Gita: the Path of Inaction-in-Action.

"There is a certain kind of action that leads to freedom and fulfillment," Krishna begins. "A certain kind of action that is always aligned with our true nature." This is the *action that is motivated by dharma.* This is the action taken in the service of our sacred calling, our duty, our vocation. In dharma, it is possible to take passionate action without creating suffering. It is possible to find authentic fulfillment of all human possibilities.

Krishna—slowly, over the course of their long dialogue—will reveal the broad outlines of an exciting program, a path through the maze of the active life that will come to be called the Path of Inaction-in-Action—or *Naishkarmya-karman.* Krishna will show Arjuna a path to the authentic self through *action in the world.* Not through renunciation and withdrawal. Not through retreat—or theologizing. And not, especially, through inaction.

Here are the central pillars of the path of action—the path of karma yoga—as expounded by Krishna. Here are the keys to Inaction-in-Action:

1. Look to your dharma.
2. Do it full out!
3. Let go of the fruits.
4. Turn it over to God.

First: Discern your dharma. "Look to your own duty," says Krishna in Chapter Two. "Do not tremble before it." Discern, name, and then embrace your own dharma.

Then: Do it full out! Knowing your dharma, do it with every fiber of your being. Bring everything you've got to it. Commit yourself utterly. In this way you can live an authentically passionate life, and you can transform desire itself into a bonfire of light.

Next: Let go of the outcome. "Relinquish the fruits of your actions," says Krishna. Success and failure in the eyes of the world are not your concern. "It is better to fail at your own dharma than to succeed at the dharma of someone else," he says.

Finally: Turn your actions over to God. "Dedicate your actions to me," says Krishna. All true vocation arises in the stream of love that flows between the individual soul and the divine soul. All true dharma is a movement of the soul back to its Ground.

Over the course of the next seventeen chapters of the Gita, Krishna carefully expounds this doctrine.

When he hears of it, Arjuna perks up. Perhaps there is a way out of this quagmire. He sits facing Krishna. And they begin to talk. From these positions, our two protagonists begin the "wondrous and holy dialogue" that will comprise the remainder of the Bhagavad Gita. The impending battle of Kurukshetra quickly recedes from view, and the narrator shines his light exclusively on the vivid conversation between these two friends.

Throughout the remaining 700 stanzas, Krishna sings his song of love, sacrifice, duty, fulfillment, and enlightened action. And Arjuna sings back—most often a song of fear, confusion, doubt, ambivalence and delusion. And we, sitting on the sidelines, and overhearing their conversation through the grace of Sanjaya, the narrator, are at times enthralled, bored, puzzled, furious, uncomprehending—but finally, enlightened.

PART II

The First Pillar:
"Look to Your Dharma"

Krishna's first practical teaching to Arjuna is simple and direct: "Arjuna, look to your dharma."

Look to your dharma!

And what is this dharma that can save Arjuna?

The Sanskrit word "dharma," as used in the Bhagavad Gita, is so full of meaning that it is impossible to grasp its full scope through any single English translation. "Dharma" can be variously, but incompletely, translated as "religious and moral law," "right conduct," "sacred duty," "path of righteousness," "true nature," and "divine order."

René Guénon, in his classic *Introduction to the Study of Hindu Doctrines,* comes as close as any author to the meaning of dharma as we will use it here. "Dharma," he says, "is the essential nature of a being, comprising the sum of its particular qualities or characteristics, and determining, by virtue of the tendencies or dispositions it implies, the manner in which this being will conduct itself, either in a general way or in relation to each particular circumstance." The word dharma in this teaching, then, refers to the *peculiar and idiosyncratic qualities of each being*—those very essential and particular qualities that make it somehow *itself.*

Scientists now tell us that every brain is like a fingerprint—utterly unique. So, too, every nervous system has its own complex idiosyncrasy, every human mind, every human body, every spirit. We might say that every person's dharma is like an internal fingerprint. It is the subtle interior blueprint of a soul.

And how precisely do we discern this dharma hidden in our being as a kind of seed? How do we manifest this unique dharma DNA?

In many cases, perhaps even in most cases, the discernment of dharma is a difficult, even agonizing process. It is only born out of our wrestling matches with doubt, with conflict, and with despair. And so, the authors of the Gita have placed their protagonist—the exemplar of the seeker of dharma—on a field of battle. The stakes are high. The decisions are complex. There are countless moral gray areas. And yet, there is no escape from choice and action.

Will Arjuna's story help us extract ourselves from our own particular quagmire of dharma? At the beginning of our encounter with the Gita, it may not be perfectly clear how much we can identify with Arjuna. We almost immediately face a small speed bump. In an outward sense, indeed, Arjuna's dilemmas around dharma seem quite different from ours. Arjuna's dharma was, of course, prescribed for him. In the caste system of ancient India, roles and dharmas were prescribed at birth. Arjuna was born into the warrior class. So, he was destined to be a warrior. It was his sacred duty to fight a just war. He never had any choice in the matter, nor was his dharma based on any particular personal qualities. Indeed, in the traditional culture in which Arjuna lived there was no such thing as a personal self. The self was a "socially embedded self." So there was no notion of *personal* dharma.

We live in a different kind of culture, of course, in which there *is* most emphatically a personal self, and therefore a personal dharma. Strangely, however, when we drill down into this issue, we discover that our dharmas, too, are in many ways not personal. They are not, in the ways that really count, our own choice—not based on our own ideas, wishes, or concepts. They are based, as Arjuna's was, on what is already mysteriously within us at birth: our fingerprint.

Krishna, in his teaching to Arjuna, points to a truth that also holds true for us.

You cannot be anyone you want to be.

You cannot be anyone you want to be?

Really?

The notion that we can be anyone we want to be is a slippery half-truth that saturates contemporary culture—reinforced by several generations of self-help literature. How many times have we heard it: "You can do anything you set your mind to."

Krishna would say, "Well, not exactly." Yes, our inner possibilities are fantastic beyond imagining. But no, these possibilities are not nearly as subject to our ego's manipulation as we might like to think. Actually, you can only expect a fulfilling life if you dedicate yourself to finding out who you *are*. To finding the ineffable, idiosyncratic seeds of possibility already planted inside. There is some surrender required here.

Thomas Merton came to precisely this conclusion after decades of spiritual practice. He wrote: "Every man has a vocation to be someone: but he must understand clearly that in order to fulfill this vocation he can only be one person: himself." This quote is enshrined as the Epigraph to this book—and for a good reason. Its wisdom is at the very heart of dharma.

So how *do* we discern our dharma? How do we discover the magnificent inner blueprint?

In the next section of the book, we will turn our attention to these very questions—to the discernment of dharma—and in particular to three important principles that can be found deep in the center of Krishna's teaching for discerning the hidden and at times inscrutable dharma within:

1. Trust in the gift.
2. Think of the small as large.
3. Listen for the call of the times.

In our narrative we will examine six stories in the light of these principles: three "great" lives, and three (so-called) "ordinary" lives. We will look at the stories of Dame Jane Goodall, one of the world's most distinguished primatologists and conservationists; we'll examine the life of Henry David Thoreau, perhaps America's most important philosopher and naturalist—himself a devotee of the Bhagavad Gita; and finally, we will take a close look at the dharma-struggles of Walt Whitman, one of America's first thoroughly American poets. Each of these human beings struggled hard with the questions of identifying and bringing forth *what was within* in ways that might illumine our own struggles. We will look, too, at three ordinary lives. We will follow the progress of our friends Katherine, Brian, and Ellen in the light of Krishna's teaching. How do they work out the realization of their true selves—the discovery of their own particular dharma?

TWO

Jane Goodall: Trust in the Gift

As a kid I was puzzled by my older brother Randy. We were only two years apart in age, we grew up with the same parents, in the same house, in the same town—and yet he seemed to inhabit an entirely different world than I. Randy loved machines. In fact, he was a genius of the technical realm. This marked him as a bewildering anomaly in our family of hopeless technophobes. Where had he come from?

When Randy was fourteen, he built his own go-cart out of scraps that were just hanging around the garage, and a discarded engine he bought at a junkyard. Randy worked on his exotic contraption intently— seriously—for hours at a time, and then roared off in a cloud of dust down the long gravel road behind our house in small-town Ohio. Jeesh. Where did this love of machines come from? Neither of my parents knew which end of a spark plug was up. Nor did any of our extended family. All clueless. Was he adopted?

Randy also had a hydroplane, an awkward homemade affair that he—with measured tinkering—made go faster than any other boat on the lake where we spent our summers. And when my uncle bought an old European sports car, Randy knew how to drive it without prior instruction. He would glide smoothly through the gears with the precision of a test pilot. Huh? How on earth did he know how to do that? Sitting confidently at the steering wheel, he would turn to me with passion in his eyes: "Wanna drive it?" I looked back blankly.

With the perspective of adulthood, I have at last found words to describe what had been happening: Randy had a gift. A freely given, mysterious aptitude for the world of the machine.

Well, I had gifts, too, and Randy, I learned later, was just as puzzled by *my* gifts as I was by his. Apparently he was especially awed by my gift for music. Even at six, I was able to sit down at my grandfather's old upright piano and pick out a tune. Later, with no training at all, I began to add harmonies, and eventually could spin out most any song I heard, playing, as my parents called it, "by ear." In all honesty, I myself sometimes marveled at this.

Gifts. Each of us has them. There is no point trying to account for them. Their source is as much a mystery as anything else in life. Nonetheless they're real—and remarkably easy to identify, even from a young age. If asked, any of us could easily name the gifts of most anyone we're close to.

Strangely, as kids, no one helped either Randy or me to understand the nature of our gifts. They were commented upon, of course. Some small attention was paid. I was given piano lessons (in a manner of speaking) with old Mrs. Croft across the street. Randy got a lame box of tools ("a boy's first tool kit") for Christmas. But no one ever suggested how important our gifts really were. No one suggested that I might want to be a pianist. Or my brother a race-car driver. My parents, and the rest of the world, seemed to have other plans for us—plans that had little to do with our idiosyncratic fascinations. We assumed that that was the way life was. No one suggested that a go-cart or an old baby grand piano were for us among the few authentic doorways into the possibility of a fulfilling and useful life. Or into the very nature of life itself. Or into our connection with God.

This may be one reason I today find the Bhagavad Gita so compelling. Here is an ancient treatise whose primary intent is to make an explicit connection between gifts and fulfillment. Between the go-cart and God.

Said Krisha to Arjuna, "It is better to fail at your own dharma than to succeed at the dharma of someone else."

Better to fail at your own dharma? Better to fail at the pursuit of one's own puny inner genius than to succeed in any other, however exalted?

Better to find your own inner fingerprint, no matter what the outcome? Really that important?

Krishna teaches Arjuna that our gifts are *sva dharma*—literally, "one's *own* dharma." Yoga sages later went on to teach that *sva dharma,* your own dharma, is equivalent to *sva bhava,* your *own being.* These gifts are somehow close to the very center of who we are.

As kids, Randy and I *almost* knew this. The go-cart and the piano were doorways into our own true natures. Full of infinite potential. They were possibility itself.

I say *almost* knew it, because we only knew it energetically—in the secret and ineffable places kids know these things. But this energetic knowing, this connection to the aliveness of the gift, is a very tender plant, as fragile as any unrooted sprout.

Don't get me wrong: The Gift itself is indestructible. "Fire cannot burn it," Krishna teaches. But the connection to the gift? The trust in the gift? The faith in the gift? This trust is, at least early on, exquisitely fragile. It is vulnerable to all manner of disruption. And here, very early, is precisely where doubt enters in. Doubt: The paralyzing affliction.

Randy and I were typical kids growing up in America in the fifties and sixties. We were sons of an ordinary middle-class family. There was very little money—but there was lots of education. And yet there was precious little faith in, or acknowledgment of, these mysteries. So our trust in The Gift was not nurtured. Indeed, at times it was run roughshod over—unknowingly.

Like most everyone else in our culture, Randy's life, and my own, would then become one long pilgrimage to regain any thin wisp of trust—to reclaim our trust in The Gift and even to turn this wily filament into a small oak of faith. We would search for a way to reestablish *faith in the way things are.*

Randy did not become a race-car driver. And I did not become a concert pianist. Would we have been happier, more fulfilled, if we had? Who knows. There are no easy formulas for these things. It's important to remember that The Gift is not itself dharma. It is only, as the old saying goes, a finger pointing to the dharma.

On the other hand, Randy does work for a large trucking company—still living close to the almighty engine (though he works as a manager in the human resources department). And I've schlepped a piano around with me from house to house my entire adult life. I still play Beethoven and Bach and Cole Porter songs in the evening, and sometimes when no one is home I accompany myself as I sing Puccini arias (very badly) to myself.

I've had moments when I felt that I was living perfectly aligned with my dharma. When the spine of life has seemed absolutely aligned. Nonetheless, I still wonder about this at times. What would my life have looked like today if my musical gift had been named, valued, nurtured, prized—really seen for what it was? In my work with young musicians at Kripalu, I have occasionally sat down at the piano to accompany a singer, or play some chamber music with a group of students. After one of these sessions—when a group of us was playing the achingly beautiful songs of Richard Strauss—one of the young violinists turned to me and said, with obvious surprise, "That was really impressive." I almost hate to admit it to myself, but that declaration—and that evening—remains a high point. Was it because I stepped for a moment back onto the road not taken?

Are there roads not taken that occasionally light you up? Do you ever fantasize about what might have been had it all gone differently?

Let's look at the question from another perspective: Do you know anyone whose gifts *were* seen, mirrored, prized? Who took the obvious road early? And thrived?

It does happen. There are people all around us who have been the recipient of this grace.

— 2 —

Dame Jane Goodall is a svelte, girlish-looking woman with beautiful eyes, a soft smile, and a quietly aristocratic bearing. She is one of the world's leading primatologists. Motivated by her love of animals (recognized, I hasten to say, when she was practically still a baby), Goodall spent decades observing the behavior of chimpanzees in Tanzania. Her remarkable fifty-year trek in the jungles of East Africa transformed our view of the primate world.

I have been fascinated by this woman for years. When I first heard her speak, I couldn't get over the fact that this sweet, velvet woman challenged the entire scientific establishment and won. (I thought of the teaching from the *Tao te Ching:* "The gentlest thing in the world overcomes the hardest thing in the world.") Goodall did not play by the rules: She *named* her chimps, for goodness' sake—the subjects of her study. She fell in love with them. And as a result, she was probably the first human being to be admitted into a roaming, in-the-jungle chimp society.

Goodall was the first scientist to document chimpanzees making tools. Not just *using* tools, but actually *making* tools. Until this discovery, tool making had been seen as *the* quintessentially human behavior: *man the toolmaker.* Goodall changed all that. She also documented chimpanzees' exhibition of what we think of as the exclusively human traits of altruism and compassion. As it turns out, chimps appear to love and care for one another. Her observations revolutionized our view of the animal world, and challenged the scientific community to reconsider well-accepted definitions of "being human." Did you know that chimpanzees' DNA differs from human DNA by a mere one percent? This has been hard for some people to accept.

Goodall's gifts have proliferated into a bonfire of contributions to the world, and have earned her many honors. She was named Dame Commander of the Order of the British Empire in a ceremony at Buckingham Palace in 2004. In recent years, Goodall has become one of the world's leading conservationists, and a champion for many aspects of the endangered natural world, particularly rain forests, primates, and other animal species. Her life, as she herself describes it in her autobiography, *Reason for Hope: A Spiritual Journey,* is one of fulfillment—an exuberant connection with the natural world, and with God. Not a perfect life: She has had her share of tragedy. Her first marriage—to the elegant Baron Hugo van Lawick—was unhappy and ended in divorce. Her second ended with the tragic death of her much-loved husband, Derek Bryceson. But still, she has (if anyone has) lived an impassioned human existence.

What is most interesting for our story is the way in which Goodall *got* to this passionate life. How did she develop from a little girl born into an aristocratic family in the heart of London to a fearless champion of the wildness of Africa? How did the little girl—who at age eighteen months collected worms in the city and took them to bed with her—become a Dame Commander of the Order of the British Empire?

The answers to these question are, of course, complex. But there is one dramatic fact of Goodall's early life that we must examine in depth here: As a child, her gifts were *named, celebrated, cherished, and nurtured.*

— 3 —

From an early age, Jane was drawn to animals and to the natural world. Here, in an excerpt from her autobiography, she recounts a tale of her life as a four-year-old on the family farm in the English countryside.

> One of my tasks was to collect the hens' eggs. As the days passed, I became more and more puzzled. Where on a chicken was there an opening big enough for an egg to come out? Apparently no one explained this properly, so I must have decided to find out for myself. I followed a hen into one of the little wooden henhouses— but of course, as I crawled after her she gave horrified squawks and hurriedly left. My young brain must have then worked out that I would have to be there first. So I crawled into another hen-house and waited, hoping a hen would come in to lay. And there I remained, crouched silently in one corner, concealed in some straw, waiting.

Jane then—at four years of age, mind you—waited patiently for hours, simply observing what was happening with the bird. Meanwhile, outside the henhouse, her family was in a panic. Where was Baby Jane? Jane continues her narration:

> At last, a hen came in, scratched about in the straw, and settled herself on her makeshift nest just in front of me. I must have kept very still or she would have been disturbed. Presently the hen half stood and I saw a round white object gradually protruding from the feathers between her legs. Suddenly with a plop, the egg

landed on the straw. With clucks of pleasure the hen shook her feathers, nudged the egg with her beak, and left. It is quite extraordinary how clearly I remember that whole sequence of events.

What comes next is important. Jane had been missing for over four hours. The household had taken to search-and-rescue mode. Excited, Jane rushed out of the henhouse, eager to tell her story. When her mother, Vanne, saw Jane, she rushed to her.

. . . despite her worry, when Vanne [Jane's mother] saw the excited little girl rushing toward the house, she did not scold me. She noticed my shining eyes and sat down to listen to the story of how a hen lays an egg: the wonder of that moment when the egg finally fell to the ground.

Where in the world did this mother come from? Where was the spanking I would have received—and would have thought perfectly justified?

Rather: "She noticed my shining eyes."

Children cannot understand the full import of The Gift. They can only feel their spirit leap up toward their object of interest—can only feel the delightful energy of fascination and enthusiasm (from the root *en theos,* literally, "the God within"). Until we develop true introspection and reflective intelligence in our teens, we cannot put these gifts into any kind of perspective at all. Only later, with the development of a mature, observing ego can we assess the kinds of potential these gifts have within them.

So, early on, these gifts must be *seen and reflected by an intelligence that has such perspective.* Trust in The Gift must be nurtured by parents, teachers, friends. The moment must not pass by unnoticed. We must be encouraged to identify with our gifts. We rely on others to see our shining eyes. Without this mirroring, we cannot understand the meaning or import of our fascination.

By the time she was four years old, Jane's gift for animals had already been seen. Named. Celebrated. Jane began to develop trust in The Gift. And only this kind of trust will allow us to learn to take risks in pursuit of The Gift—risks that will often be required in the expression of dharma.

Said Jane as an adult, "I was lucky to be provided with a mother wise enough to nurture and encourage my love of living things and my passion for knowledge."

This is a whopping understatement. It gets better. The very same brilliant mom—Vanne—followed Jane into the wilds of Tanzania and supported her, kept house for her (rather, "kept hut for her") as she developed her first jungle station to work with chimpanzees. A native Tanzanian forest ranger, upon first meeting these two women fresh off the boat, "assumed," reflects Jane, "upon depositing these two crazy Englishwomen at their first camp that they would pull up stakes within a few weeks."

"Little did they know," said Jane.

Who does not read in amazement the account of Vanne, deep in middle age, trekking to Tanzania, and living in a precarious and frightening lakeside camp (later there was mass murder just across the lake) while her daughter spent nights alone in the jungle with the chimps? Crazy Englishwomen.

Vanne not only felt compelled to reflect Jane's gift to her. She felt *a responsibility to The Gift.* I suspect that Vanne had not read the Bhagavad Gita, but there she would have found this very teaching. We have a responsibility to The Gift. The Gift is God in disguise.

In Jane Goodall we have a fairly uncommon example of a life in which just about everything was working to support dharma. But isn't it good to know that these things can happen? "I had a mother who not only tolerated but also encouraged my passion for nature and animals and who, even more important, taught me to believe in myself," wrote Jane.

Taught me to believe in myself.

One of the lessons of Jane's life: It only takes one person. There were not a lot of others lining up to support Jane in her decades of life with the chimps. Most saw her choices as entirely strange, and rather gave her up for good when she disappeared into the jungle at age twenty-six, not to emerge again for decades.

Jane's autobiography is a compelling catalog of the maturation of gifts. She describes how, early in her years at Gombe, she had to follow the troop of chimps through the brush for hours or days at a time to get a single chimpanzee sighting. She waited patiently with them through dark nights for almost a year before a single chimp would even come within a hundred yards of her. Her patience was a maturation of the *possibility* she exhibited back in England as a four-year-old—resolutely watching that hen.

— 4 —

Quite honestly, as I read Goodall's autobiography, I thought: Well, where was the struggle? Where was the doubt? I wanted to know what she left out. Those would have been the good parts, I thought. I really had trouble believing her story could be that good. But then I realized: This is what a life of certitude looks like. Rather than conflict and drama, all of Goodall's energy went into her creativity, until finally she ignited into that bonfire of contribution to the world. Jane's experience is what we might call the Direct Path to Dharma. It can happen. It is magnificent when it does.

But my observation leads me to believe that Goodall's story is the exception rather than the rule. As a person who has taken the Indirect Path to Dharma, I long to hear another story: What happens when our gifts are not met with the same remarkable understanding and perspective that Jane encountered?

Do you remember Brian, the Catholic priest whom I introduced in Chapter One? Now here is a man with whom I can identify.

Brian is a man whose gifts were not seen or reflected to him as a child. He felt a calling to music even as a kid. When he was six, his uncle Kevin bought him a little blue plastic organ. It was for years his most precious possession (and still remains in the closet of his boyhood room). Brian soon transformed his motley crew of stuffed animals into a choir that he conducted from the little plastic bench that came with the organ. He even made himself a miniature choirmaster robe—from a yellowing sheet that he got his sister to sew. I just know his eyes were shining like crazy while he was directing that choir of bears and monkeys and giraffes. How could anyone miss that? You'd think his mother would have straightaway signed him up for choirmaster school.

But Brian's mother was not so interested in his stuffed-animal choir. She had big plans for Brian. He was going to become a priest. Every generation in her family—all the way back to Ireland—had had at least one priest, and she had no intention of being the mother who broke the tradition. It was a noble tradition; at least that's what everyone said at Sunday family dinners after church. It was good for the family, and for the Church and for the world. And it was—she lost no opportunity in saying it—her deepest wish. Brian wanted to please his mother. Enough to put himself aside?

Brian can remember the exact moment when he realized he would not be a church musician. He was fourteen. His mother was talking with pride to Uncle Kevin about Brian's eventual destiny: ". . . maybe a monsignor, or even a bishop. He has the gift." "What gift?" Brian wondered. He could feel his face redden. After a few minutes, he went to his room and cried into his pillow.

The next day—and periodically over the next year—Brian talked the situation over with Sister Mary Joseph at school. She listened sympathetically, nodding her head in its starched habit. "Now, Brian," she said with authentic kindness in her voice, which made the lesson go in deeper, "you have to understand that we don't always get what we want. This is what adulthood is all about," echoing almost perfectly Brian's mother's view. "Your mother knows more than you yet do about life. And I believe, too, that this is what God wants for you. And you know, it is very pleasing in God's eyes to be a priest. This is a gift you will give to God."

"This is what adulthood is," thought Brian. "I can do this." He felt his spine stiffen.

Brian surrendered to the call heard not by himself, but by his parents and teachers. What resulted was much more serious than anyone could have imagined. It was the silent tragedy of self-betrayal.

Remember Krishna's teaching: We cannot be anyone we want to be. We can only authentically be who we are. "The attempt to live out someone else's dharma brings extreme spiritual peril," says Krishna. *Extreme spiritual peril!*

If you bring forth what is within you it will save you. If you do not, it will destroy you.

And what, precisely, is destroyed?

Energy is destroyed first. Those shining eyes. And then faith. And then hope. And then life itself.

The increasing deadening of aliveness that Brian experienced as he went into the seminary is the very opposite of Jane Goodall's experience. When a life is founded on self-betrayal, the habit of self-betrayal proliferates until we are at peril of not remembering who we are at all. There is a slow deadening of spirit as we try to pick up the burdens of adulthood without the energy of The Gift. Our work can be motivated by obligation, by hunger for the external rewards of accomplishment, or by strongly reinforced ideas about who we should be in this lifetime. But none of these motivations has the authentic energy required for mastery of a profession. So, all of these motivations lead slowly to a downward spiral that tends to crash, as it did with Brian, at midlife. Without the balm of real fulfillment there is a growing emptiness inside. Finally, it requires a heroic effort to simply go on with life in the face of this emptiness. The light in the eyes goes out.

— 5 —

After a year or so in the jungles of Tanzania, Jane began to make thrilling contact with her chimpanzees. In *Reason for Hope,* she describes an extraordinary meeting of minds between chimpanzee and scientist—a meeting for which her henhouse experience had prepared her—and a meeting that would change her view of the possibilities of her work. Here she describes an early moment with David Greybeard, a gray-chinned male chimp who became her first real "friend" in the troop:

> "As David [the chimp] and I sat there, I noticed a ripe red fruit from an oil nut palm lying on the ground. I held it toward him on the palm of my hand. David glanced at me and reached to take the nut. He dropped it, but gently held my hand. I needed no words to understand his message of reassurance: he didn't want

the nut, but he understood my motivation, he knew I meant well. To this day I remember the soft pressure of his fingers."

As Jane made more frequent connections with the objects of her fascination, she describes an increasing sense of *knowing her dharma*. "More and more often," she says, "I found myself thinking, 'This is where I belong. This is what I came into this world to do.'"

In her sixties and seventies, Jane became a world traveler and lecturer, urging human beings everywhere to widen their circle of compassion to include the animal world.

She describes the maturation of her sense of dharma. "Each one of us matters, has a role to play, and makes a difference," she says. She describes hearing a "still small voice" that guides her, and that she believes to be the "Voice of God." She says, "Of course, it is usually called the voice of conscience, and if we feel more comfortable with that definition, that's fine. Whatever we call it, the important thing, I think, is to try to do what the voice tells us."

And then Jane sounds a note that is a theme throughout this book. As her connection to her dharma matures, she increasingly has a sense that she is not the doer of her actions, but that God is working through her. "I always have this feeling—which may not be true at all—that I am being used as a messenger. There are times before a lecture when I have been absolutely exhausted, or actually sick, and terrified that I am going to utterly fail the audience. And those lectures are often among the best. Because, I think, I have been able to tap into the spiritual power that is always there, providing strength and courage if only we reach out."

—— 6 ——

Henry David Thoreau said, "The youth gets together his materials to build a bridge to the moon, or, perchance, a palace or temple on the earth, and, at length, the middle-aged man concludes to build a woodshed with them."

For Brian, at midlife, even building a woodshed would have been a stretch. By the time he was forty-five, he was depressed. Being a priest required a heroic effort for him: mammoth amounts of self-will; a good deal of posing; and always having to bear the palpable absence of true mastery. True mastery, authentic dharma, is not possible without the kernel of The Gift at the center.

Psychologists call this inner and outer poseur the "false self." The name says it all. The false self is a collection of ideas we have in our minds about who we *should* be. Sometimes these ideas—most often planted in childhood—can be so strong that they override our capacity to see who we actually are, or at least to fully embrace it. They become a kind of learning disability. Our capacity to see the world clearly is thwarted.

Brian is an exemplar of the quiet suffering of the false self: There develops a stilted relationship to work: mediocrity, lack of interest, lack of enthusiasm, lack of soul-connection to work. This eventually begins to invade even the sphere of play, for as Thoreau said, famously, "Play comes after work."

But there is something resilient about gifts: Their light is never fully extinguished. Our gifts are so close to the core of our being that they can never really be entirely destroyed, no matter how deadening the life. My brother still has two motorcycles that he rides in his spare time, a truck, and a BMW. He did not become a race-car driver, but he does go to Germany in the summer to a motorcycle-riding school in the Alps. Shining eyes, still.

Brian discovered deep in midlife that his gift of music was still calling out to him from someplace deep inside. Along with it there was a growing ache. And a growing unwillingness to live out the rest of his days without going for it. The older he got, the less able he was to maintain the ruse of the false self. As we get deeper into life, we become more aware of life's finitude. We discover the truth taught by Krishna: You cannot be anyone you want to be. Your one and only shot at a fulfilled life is being yourself—whoever that is.

Furthermore, at a certain age it finally dawns on us that, shockingly, no one really *cares* what we're doing with our life. This is a most unsettling discovery to those of us who have lived someone else's dream and eschewed our own: *No one really cares except us.* When you scratch the surface, you finally discover that it doesn't really matter a whit who else you disappoint if you're disappointing yourself. The only question that makes sense to ask is: Is your life working for you?

For Brian, at forty-five and deep into another career, the first step was to develop a process through which he could face the truth. He was so unhappy with his life as a priest that he had been on antidepressants for almost five years. Finally, out of desperation, he got into psychotherapy. There, he allowed himself to face his suffering—and finally, to name The Gift.

With the naming came a flood of regret. It was not the tidal wave of hope and relief he had counted on. Learning to embrace The Gift at midlife is complicated. Because naming The Gift and celebrating it also mean grieving for lost opportunities. They mean facing squarely the suffering of self-betrayal.

The deeper we get into life, the more difficult it can be to make the commitment to The Gift. Other commitments have to be relinquished. Space has to be made. Not only that, but Brian was terrified that, having carved out space, he might fail at his expression of The Gift. And indeed, there are no guarantees. Perhaps he would be a truly lousy—or even unhappy—church musician. Was he willing to take the risk? Willing to jettison all he had worked for?

There is no way around it: Dharma always involves, at some point, a leap off a cliff in the dark. Jane Goodall made her leaps early in life—and with a good deal of support. Still, there were leaps. Still, there was plenty of dark. What is most inspiring about Goodall's life is the way in which she developed *a faith in the leap itself.*

Did Brian leap? Or stay rooted to the edge of the cliff? We will follow his progress later on in our story.

THREE

Henry David Thoreau:
Think of the Small as Large

"Be resolutely and faithfully what you are," wrote Henry David Thoreau. "Be humbly what you aspire to be . . . man's noblest gift to man is his sincerity, for it embraces his integrity also."

There is no greater champion of dharma in American letters than Henry David Thoreau, and he is one of the few who actually used the word "dharma" in his writing and in his thought. Thoreau was an American poet, naturalist, surveyor, philosopher, and a leading Transcendentalist. He is best known for his masterpiece, *Walden,* and for his essay *Civil Disobedience.* These, and his many other works, have inspired some of the world's greatest exemplars of freedom—giants like Mahatma Gandhi, Martin Luther King Jr., and Nelson Mandela.

As it turns out, America's greatest natural philosopher was also a student of the Bhagavad Gita. He studied it—along with his mentor, Ralph Waldo Emerson—and often quoted from the majestic 1785 translation by Charles Wilkins. The Gita was one of the books Thoreau most prized during his two-and-a-half-year adventure at Walden Pond. Sitting at the side of Walden watching a sunrise, he would at times imagine himself as a yogi from ancient times absorbed in contemplation. "Depend upon it," he wrote in a letter to his friend H.G.O. Blake, "that rude and careless as I am, I would fain practice the yoga faithfully."

Like every good yogi, Thoreau saw his entire life as a kind of trek toward dharma. "A man tracks himself through life," he wrote. "One should be always on the trail of one's own deepest nature. For it is the fearless living out of your own essential nature that connects you to the Divine." He often quotes the Gita to himself in his personal journals, especially Krishna's counsel about dharma: "A man's own calling," he lets Krishna remind him, "with all its faults, ought not to be forsaken."

Unlike Jane Goodall, young Thoreau was not a celebrity in his own day. Far from it. He was widely seen as "an irresponsible idler, a trial to his family, and no credit to his town" (to quote one of his grumpy Concord neighbors). In short, Thoreau was seen as a loser.

I fell in love with Thoreau in graduate school. I loved how this guy had apparently embraced his inner loser. I had secretly felt like something of a loser myself, especially during the tormented social maneuvering of high school. But I had no idea there would be power in *embracing* this position on the social chessboard. I thought this side of me was to be hidden at all costs. So I tried all the harder to be seen as one of the elect: the winners.

Thoreau, known today as one of America's greatest writers, was widely disregarded, overlooked, and scoffed at in his own time. His first book, *A Week on the Concord and Merrimack Rivers,* never sold even the small, thousand-copy print run of its first edition. *Walden,* his masterpiece— now read by virtually every college sophomore—languished on bookstore shelves for years. Indeed, the first edition of 2,000 copies took eight years to sell, and there wasn't a second printing until just before Thoreau's untimely death in 1862.

Thoreau's resolutely unconventional life as the mystic of Concord required a different kind of courage than did Goodall's. It required the courage to acknowledge The Gift in the face of widespread disapprobation. It required the resilience to breathe air in the same town in which he was seen as a kind of community joke. And it required Thoreau to develop a fierce sense of autonomy. As a result of his steadfast loyalty to his gifts, of course, the world came to respect them as well. And that same scoffing world has now been applauding his genius—and his gritty aphorisms—for over a hundred and fifty years.

—— 2 ——

Thoreau did come to value The Gift. But he made one largely unknown and yet fascinating stab at "fitting in" early on in his life—one attempt to be who he thought he *should* be rather than who he *was*. I find it strangely reassuring to examine this anomalous chapter in his life.

In May of 1843, at the age of twenty-six, Henry David Thoreau set off for New York City. He was intent on securing his place in the city's sparkling literary scene. Thoreau had already begun to find his footing as a writer. He'd discovered that he was not, as he had thought, a poet, but a prose artist. By the time he left for New York, his prose had already matured beyond the influence of his highly respected teacher, Ralph Waldo Emerson. (Thoreau was aware that Emerson was not happy with his prose, and to his way of thinking, this proved only that he was indeed moving in the right direction—toward himself.) By May of 1843, just several years out of Harvard and with only a slim body of work under his belt, Thoreau nonetheless judged himself ready to mingle with the great and near-great of the American world of letters—Horace Greeley, Henry James Sr., W. H. Channing.

Thoreau was a colossal failure in the city. But the story of this failure, and of Thoreau's thirteen months in New York, is revealing. It shows the unconventional nature lover attempting to develop a writing career *in the conventional way*. He was not well accepted by the New York literary world, which saw him as impossibly rough-hewn and ordinary. He *was* rough-hewn, of course. Nathaniel Hawthorne describes his face: "Thoreau is as ugly as sin, long-nosed, queer-mouthed, and with uncouth and rustic, though courteous, manners, corresponding very well with such an exterior." Thoreau himself laughingly commented on his beak of a nose, which he called "my most prominent feature." But Hawthorne (who was himself supremely handsome) adds an important modifier to his description: ". . . his ugliness is of an honest and agreeable fashion, and becomes him much better than beauty."

Thoreau tried to sparkle in the literary salons of New York. The attempt fell flat. He tried to style his prose to appeal to the fashions of the day. His work was mediocre—and widely disregarded. Throughout his entire year in New York, Thoreau never managed to publish more than one slim book review, in spite of his powerful determination to be published with the big boys. Eventually, toward the end of his stay, the pain of rejection forced him to reach even more deeply into his own unique gift. Who am I? What is my voice? What do I have to say? Digging down into his own inner world, and longing for his roots in the woods of Concord, Thoreau—from his tenement in New York—wrote the brilliant sketch on "the first sparrow of spring," which would become one of the most famous passages in *Walden*. (As it turns out, an overwhelming amount of great nature writing has been written in the city by writers who long for their true homes.)

Finally, the unhappy writer—floundering, separated from himself—had to go home, tail between his legs. He returned to Concord—to his woods, to his pond, to his father's pencil factory, and to Emerson's house. "Be humbly who you are," he wrote upon arriving home.

Thoreau's failure in New York was a life lesson. *Be who you are. Do what you love. Follow your own distant drummer.* "A man's own calling ought not to be forsaken!"

Failure is a part of all great dharma stories. And great dharma failures do not just happen early in life. They routinely happen throughout life. We only know who we are by trying on various versions of ourselves. We try various dharmas on to see if they fit. How do I look in this? Yes, this looks cool, and feels great. Or: egad, no! Not in a million years. When the clothes don't fit well, it clarifies things for us. In any quest for dharma there will inevitably be lots of trying on of outfits.

Thoreau's failure is particularly instructive, because it emerged from a dharma error most of us have made at one point or another in our lives: the attempt to be *big*. The attempt to be, in fact, bigger than we *are*. A confusion about the right size of a life of dharma.

—— 3 ——

Remember Ellen—my friend the psychiatric nurse?

Ellen, as you recall, was in a muddle about her calling. Any of her friends could see that she had been acting from the center of her dharma for years. Even complete strangers could see it. But she saw it only fleetingly. She had never fully named her dharma, accepted it, embraced it.

As a result, she had gone through too many years feeling that she had somehow not entirely won at the game of life.

Much of Ellen's muddle was in her *thinking about her dharma.* She thought that her job, her calling, was *too small.* It didn't match up to her fantasies of what a calling *should be.*

Some of her thinking, no doubt, was inspired by the views of our culture about nursing. Caretaking roles are not highly regarded by our society, to say the least. The nobility of the helping professions is all too invisible. Nurses are taken for granted—and doctors are too often esteemed not because they are wonderful caretakers but because they are good businesspeople. (Ellen, by the way, has no problem with her self-esteem in the face of doctors. For thirty years she has presided—day in and day out—over an enormously complex psych unit through which doctors merely cruised from time to time.)

But Ellen's problems started long before her nursing career. I had known Ellen's parents—both now long dead—and I knew how some of their ideas had inevitably found their way into Ellen's head. Ellen's father, Bud, was caught between the twin agonies of grandiosity and devaluing. He was a bright, entrepreneurial man, who had tried to create a business selling frozen cookies long before frozen foods were a staple of American life. His ideas were innovative and really quite brilliant, but a hairsbreadth before their time. He would have made a fortune had he tried them out a few years later. Bud's business venture failed, and he remained caught for the rest of his career directing a school lunch program, which seemed to him a real betrayal of his potential.

By the time I knew him, Bud felt defeated. He was cynical about work, and obsessed with security, safety, and keeping expectations low. Shortly after I graduated from college he suggested that I might consider driving a truck for a living, because it was a safe and steady income. "You'll never go hungry," he said. He had himself tasted hunger: While Bud was perfecting the frozen cookie, his family had endured several bleak winters in a house they came to call "Hungry Hill."

Ellen—through Bud—had come smack up against two of the enemies of dharma: grandiosity, and its flip side, devaluing. (In short, the problem of size.) Grandiosity and devaluing both represent unrealistic thinking about possibility. Grandiosity motivates us to try to be bigger than we could possibly be. Devaluing makes us think of ourselves as smaller than we actually are.

Ellen's father often told her that his harsh discipline was "for her own good," and that it was part of a grand (his own term for it) strategy to help her make of her life "a great work of art." His precise words were devastating, and I wince when Ellen reminds me of them: "You are a piece of granite," he said to her, time and again. "I am the sculptor. And I will *grind you fine*." This was said with sadistic emphasis. "And if," he continued, working himself up into a lather, "if perchance my mallet slips and the whole thing crumbles to dust, well, *I will take that chance*."

This young woman didn't have a prayer. Nursing—for which she was in every single way suited—did not in her eyes really qualify her life as "a work of art." So Ellen remained split—as her father was—between big ideas and what seemed to be an unacceptably smaller reality. For obvious reasons, Ellen could not always embrace who *she actually was*. So she lived with doubt—sometimes unsure about what otherwise could have been embraced as an immensely satisfying career.

The question of the "size" of a life is tricky territory, because big ideas also have an expansive quality to them that allow us to experiment with who we *can* be. Big ideas are not bad. But somehow, the bigness must remain closer to the ground than it did for Ellen's father. The bigness, must, in fact, come *through the smallness*. Thoreau discovered this on his trek to New York.

"Be resolutely and faithfully what you are," said Thoreau—not who you think you should be. Thoreau's early struggle was to be "right-sized." Not too big, not too small. It was his resolute embrace of a right-sized self that became for him the doorway into a full life.

Having landed back on both feet at Walden Pond, Thoreau said, "I would rather walk to Rutland [Vermont] than to Jerusalem." This was written at a time when there was much grand gesturing about the metaphysical Jerusalem. No grand gesture for Thoreau. No Jerusalem. Gritty (and nearby) Vermont would do.

"Think of the small as large," wrote Lao Tzu, the author of the *Tao te Ching*. Thoreau is the great American genius of this aphorism. *Think of the small as large*. "See yourself as a grain of sand," suggests Chögyam

Trungpa, the Tibetan crazy-wisdom guru, "see yourself as the smallest of the small. Then you can make room for the whole world."

— 4 —

By May of 1845, Thoreau was home from New York City and back in the woods at Walden Pond—building his cabin. His feet were solidly planted back on *terra firma*. He was engaged in dharma that was right-sized. Thoreau now saw clearly that the journey of a writer was not the outer journey to New York, but the inner journey to his own voice. He was going to be himself, and to hell with the naysayers. He would live out the Transcendentalist view that "human nature in general is revealed to each person through his own nature in particular." *His own nature in particular.* Walden Pond was where Henry David Thoreau would intentionally conduct this inner journey to himself.

At this crossroads in his life something fascinating happens to Thoreau: His powers as a writer explode. Two days after moving to Walden Pond, he wrote a lengthy entry in his journal about his personal experience of "self-emancipation." He was exploring the idea of an exhilarating personal freedom in a passage in which he had been referring to the West Indies. He wrote, "Self-emancipation in the West Indies of a man's thinking and imagining provinces . . . should be more than his island territory. *One emancipated heart and intellect! It would knock the fetters from a million slaves.*"

After the emptiness (and "insincerity") of his New York experience comes a freedom at Walden Pond so big it can *knock the fetters from a million slaves.* As young Thoreau connected once again to himself, he felt reunited with the world, and he saw clearly the relationship between his own freedom and the freedom of the world. Mahatma Gandhi would make the same discovery, imprisoned in India just a hundred years later. And Nelson Mandela's resolute and resilient inner freedom—even while in shackles—finally did in fact liberate millions. Both Gandhi and Mandela were dedicated readers of Thoreau.

Thoreau discovered the intimate connection between the *individual* and the *field*—between the particular and the universal, between the small and the large. This was a central principle of the Transcendentalists. But Thoreau had not fully grasped it until now. It was an insight that would emerge directly from his newfound faith in authenticity. Thoreau now wrote excitedly in his journal, "The whole is in each man."

The mystic relationship of the individual to the universal is absolutely central to the wisdom of the Bhagavad Gita, and we will be hearing it played as a central theme in Krishna's teachings. But interestingly, before the principle was given its definitive explication in the Bhagavad Gita, it was the centerpiece of one of the most ancient dharma tales in the Indian oral-wisdom tradition. This is the wonderful story of Indra's Net—a tale Thoreau and Emerson almost certainly knew. It is the most pointed ancient investigation of the relationship between the small and the large.

—— 5 ——

Indra was "the thunderbolt God"—the greatest god in the ancient Vedic pantheon, which emerged at the dawn of yoga metaphysics in India at least 3,000 years ago. Indra lived (word had it) in the clouds at the peak of Mount Meru—the most sacred mountain of the Hindu tradition. Meru is considered the center of the world in Vedic cosmology, what Joseph Campbell sometimes referred to as the *axis mundi,* or "the immoveable spot." Just the place for a great god to reside.

Around his celestial home Indra had flung a vast net—a web stretching out infinitely in all directions. Each vertex, or node, of this net was held together by a glittering jewel. There were infinite nodes, and so there were infinite jewels.

What does it mean? Just this: Each gem in the net represents a human soul. And though each of these jewels is unique (has its own fingerprint!) it also reflects in its polished surface the image of all the other jewels. American philosopher and psychologist Alan Watts imagined this web as a multidimensional spiderweb. He said, "Imagine this web in the early morning, covered with dewdrops. And every dewdrop contains the reflection of all the other dewdrops. And, in each reflected dewdrop, the reflections of all the other dewdrops in that reflection. And so on ad infinitum."

Each jewel in Indra's net represents both *itself* as a particular jewel, and, at the same time, the *entire web.* So, any change in one gem would be reflected in the whole. Indeed, the individual gem *is* the whole. In the words of Indologist Sir Charles Eliot, "Every object in the world is not merely itself but involves every other object and in fact IS everything else."

It is, therefore, the sacred duty of every individual human soul to be utterly and completely itself—to be *that* jewel at *that* time and in *that* place, and to be that jewel *utterly*. It is in this way—merely by being itself—that one jewel holds together its own particular corner of Space and Time. The action of each individual soul holds together the entire net. Small and large at the same time.

In another great Hindu scripture—*The Mahabharata* (the great epic poem of which the Gita is a part)—Krishna teaches about dharma: "Dharma upholds both this-worldly and other-worldly affairs," he says. Krishna here introduces a fascinating new dimension to dharma. Dharma upholds and expresses the order, harmony, and essential nature of individual beings in the world, and at the same time upholds an unseen inner world order. (It is this order and harmony that had been threatened on the field of Kurukshetra, and that could only be saved by Arjuna's faithfully playing his small role—just as Thoreau would later play his.)

Our actions in expression of our dharma—my actions, your actions, everyone's actions—are infinitely important. They connect us to the soul of the world. They create the world. Small as they may appear, they have the power to uphold the essential inner order of the world.

— 6 —

Thoreau discovered this principle through his own experience, and through his close examination of nature and of life. Sitting in the center of his own *axis mundi* at Walden, he was lit up with the energy of the cosmos. It all poured out in his writing. For two and a half years, Thoreau unleashed upon the world a torrent of words. Says his biographer Robert Richardson Jr., "[Thoreau] produced more writing of higher quality over a greater range of subjects while he was living at Walden than at any other period of his life. In twenty-six months, he wrote two complete drafts of *A Week,* a complete draft of *Walden,* a lecture on his life at Walden, a lecture essay on Thomas Carlyle, and the first third of *The Maine Woods.*"

In unleashing his own freedom, Thoreau *did* free a million slaves. He discovered that his authentic words had real power. When written from "the immoveable spot" they could, indeed, change the world. In the essay *On Civil Disobedience,* Thoreau outlined the justification for active resistance against both the immorality of slavery and the futility of America's war with Mexico. This powerful document has reverberated through history since: It directly inspired the actions of Mahatma Gandhi and Martin Luther King Jr., and Nelson Mandela. And it has inspired generations of Americans to be themselves.

The fact that Thoreau's trek to Walden was such an altogether homespun experiment makes us love him all the more. As it turns out, his exotic experiment took place a scant mile and a half from home. Recently, scholars have discovered that his mother often brought him cookies and sandwiches. His experiment was only about two steps beyond sleeping in the backyard in a tent. It was not heroic. And, of course, he never claimed that it was. It was a small act, and that smallness was the very source of its virtue—the secret source of its largeness. Later on, capturing this paradox perfectly, he would say about his inner and outer peregrinations, "I have traveled extensively in Concord."

It is fascinating to watch Thoreau at Walden Pond begin to take full ownership of his idiosyncratic rhythms. It was at Walden that he came to know and to embrace the ecology of his inner life. He spent his mornings reading the great European authors: Goethe, Carlyle, Schiller. And in the afternoons he sallied forth, "sauntering," as he said, for walks that could last well into the evening. He lived a thoughtful, intellectual life, but also an appealingly simple one. There was no attempt at heroism here. No grandiosity.

Finally, Thoreau was able to fully declare himself—to clearly name and celebrate his dharma: "I am a mystic, a Transcendentalist, and a natural philosopher to boot," he declared. It was not easy to declare oneself a mystic in nineteenth-century Concord. In most people's minds this translated directly into "loafer." Still, having claimed his dharma and having felt the power of this act, he could now give his advice with authority: "Do what you love!" he wrote exuberantly. "Know your own bone: gnaw at it, bury it, unearth it, and gnaw it still."

Know your own bone!

—— 7 ——

Ellen's task, now, at midlife, is to know her bone—her gift for care-taking. And knowing it, to see its true largeness. For that, she will need help. She will need mirroring. I try to do this for her when I can.

Recently, I went with Ellen to visit Jane, a centenarian of whom Ellen has charge. Jane lives alone—at one hundred and two years of age—in her own second-floor walk-up. This little apartment was designed and decorated sometime in the late fifties, and nothing has changed. It is fitted out with aging wall-to-wall shag carpet of an orange color that any of us who lived through the 1960s will recognize. There is the inevitable knotty pine "early American" furniture, with lots of fabric wreaths and lime-green ceramic lamps shaped like dolphins. There is the faint smell of urine. There is plenty of dust.

And there is one-hundred-and-two-year-old Jane. Puttering around in her housecoat, drinking coffee and leafing absentmindedly through a stack of papers. There on the kitchen table are her many bills—which she is obviously paying herself, thank you—and a neat list in a notebook of bills paid and unpaid. (Why do we assume that the elderly cannot do these things for themselves?)

Jane takes us for a tour of the apartment. Kitchenette. (Also knotty pine.) Bathroom. Old-person smell. Bedroom. White-painted furniture and more shag carpet—turquoise this time. While we're in the bedroom, Jane remembers something she wants to give to Ellen, and opens a top drawer of her bureau. As she does so, inexpertly, the whole bureau begins to tip in Jane's direction. Ellen flies into action. She catches the bureau in her powerful nurse's arms. She sits the shaken Jane down on the bed to make sure she is all right. Then she makes a joke of the whole thing. Fifteen minutes later, when Ellen refers to this incident, Jane says, "Well, that never happened. I don't know what you're talking about." Ellen just laughs, and opens a probiotic-rich yogurt for Jane to taste.

All the while, I'm watching Ellen. She's lit up. She's having fun. She is goofing on Jane, and on the whole scene, throughout, but in the nicest way. She is taking care of little things unobtrusively. She cleans up a spill in the bathroom. As we prepare to leave, she touches Jane tenderly, smoothing back her hair. Jane squeezes her hand. "What would I ever do without you?"

Ellen chuckles as we walk back out to the car. I observe to myself, OK, she really *is* lit up. There are the shining eyes. She is not just making this up. She's not just doing this out of obligation, or to be a good person. She genuinely likes this stuff. Taking care of Jane would make me crazy. I would be full of resentment within half an hour, and would be fantasizing about sending her off to the nursing home within two days' time.

My ongoing dialogue with Ellen has helped me to realize something: I never really liked helping, even though—strangely—I chose "the helping professions." I didn't even like that term: helping. Thoreau said: "If I knew for a certainty that a man was coming to my house with the conscious design of doing me good, I should run for my life." Yes.

But Ellen is completely herself when helping. There is none of the forced helpfulness that would characterize my efforts. This is what a real caretaker-soul looks like, I thought. This is why we all have to have different dharmas. Every base is covered somehow, but only if everyone acts on their authentic calling. Only if everyone holds together her part of the net.

On another occasion, I helped Ellen with a yard sale—schlepping mountains of tchotchkes and old furniture from the garage to the driveway, setting up long tables and hanging largely gratuitous price tags on what was now virtually junk. (Ellen didn't really want the money. She just wanted to get rid of her stuff.) I'm not sure exactly how this happened, but every other car was full of people Ellen knew. The most fun were her patients from the psych unit in the VA. Some showed up on motorcycles. Some in soft, handworked leather vests and headbands. Some in rusted-out vans—cigarettes hanging out of their mouths, and with their latest sixty-five-year-old girlfriend riding shotgun. Ellen joked with them. "Elmer, I hope to God you took your meds before you got on that bike. I mean the meds we prescribed for you, not the ones you bought on the Internet."

Since I have been writing this book, Ellen and I have been talking off and on about dharma. She said to me one day, "I think my dharma is to create a safe space for people. To create a safe container in which people can thrive and be themselves. To be a kind of home base for folks—especially those who have no other home base."

Ellen and I have created an ongoing joke. I direct The Institute for Extraordinary Living at Kripalu. We decided that Ellen's house—for many years a sanctuary for me, as for so many others—would henceforth be known as The Institute for Ordinary Living. It would be a place where I could feel both of my feet on the ground. It has been for me through the years a place where I can embrace the magic of ordinary living. Whereas my mind is often in the clouds, Ellen's is right on the ground.

And yet, in spite of all of this, deep into middle age, Ellen is still occasionally confounded by her early demons of grandiosity and devaluing. Ellen continues to wrestle with the process of naming and claiming her dharma. What is my life really about? Does my little dharma really matter? These doubts, when their tracks have been laid down early, become remarkably intractable. And they create suffering.

— 8 —

Each one of us has, at some point, been caught like Ellen between the twin perils of grandiosity and devaluing. On the one hand, we secretly daydream about being famous, being glamorous, being renowned for some great work. On the other hand, we fear that our small lives—such as they are—don't amount to a hill of beans. So there they are: the devil—grandiosity. And the deep blue sea—devaluing. They are both unhappy ways to live.

What is really the right size for our life—for our dharma? Not too big. Not too small.

In New York, Thoreau was reaching too high. He had an *idea* of greatness. But it became a rigidly held concept that disconnected him from his true greatness, which was both smaller and larger than he thought. At Walden, however, Thoreau was right-sized. At Walden he undertook just a small experiment. He was near enough to home to get his daily delivery of cookies. He was comfortable enough, yes. But he was just a little uncomfortable, too. There was a stretch. Just enough of a stretch. And right in that balance, Thoreau found the correct size for his life. And his dharma exploded with energy.

Right size is everything.

Think of the small as large.

—— FOUR ——

Walt Whitman:
Listen for the Call of the Times

The Civil War "saved" Walt Whitman. He said so himself in the waning days of his long and eventful life. How precisely it was that the war saved Whitman is one of the most compelling—and largely unknown—stories of dharma in American history. And the telling of this story gives us the opportunity to look at the third—and in many ways the most complex—hallmark of dharma-discernment: the intersection of The Gift and the The Times.

Most of us, of course, know Walt Whitman as a celebrated American poet, essayist, philosopher, and patriot. He lived from 1819 to 1892. His masterpiece, *Leaves of Grass,* has often been called the first great American epic poem. But his work was exceedingly controversial during his lifetime, and *Leaves of Grass* was widely viewed as obscene for its overt sexuality. Whitman himself was—like Thoreau—seen as a loafer, a failure, and a ne'er-do-well. And worse, in Whitman's case, a "sexual invert." "Guilty," said one reviewer of *Leaves of Grass,* "of that horrible sin not to be mentioned among Christians."

What most of us don't know is that Walt Whitman found what he believed was his truest calling, as a volunteer nurse during the Civil War. Between 1862 and the end of the war, he visited thousands of sick, wounded, lonely, and dying young men in the hospitals of the Union Army. He brought them fruit, candy, cigarettes, writing paper. But mostly he brought them himself. His tender spirit. His generous nature. His broken heart. And by the conclusion of the war, he understood that these suffering men and boys had called forth something within him more precious than even his gift for poetry.

Whitman's work in the hospitals used him up. It wore him out. It ruined his health, and initiated a slow slide toward death. But he never regretted it—or counted the cost. "I only gave myself," he told a friend. "But I got the boys."

His story shows us why it is that we cannot look at The Gift only for its own sake. The Gift cannot reach maturity until it is used in the service of a greater good. In order to ignite the full ardency of dharma, *The Gift must be put in the service of The Times.*

In the Bhagavad Gita, Arjuna finds his dharma calling him to the center of the greatest cataclysm of the age. It is no accident that the priestly authors of the Gita place their exemplar at the exact center of the suffering of the times. It is precisely Arjuna's offering of himself to the urgent call of the moment that will turn his gifts into world-transforming dharma.

If you bring forth what is within you it will save you. Yes. But this saving is not just for you. It is for the common good. If you bring forth what is within you, it will save the world. It will rescue the times. It will save the whole people. Likewise: If you do not bring forth what is within you it will destroy you. But not just you. If you do not bring forth what is within you, it will destroy the whole people.

—— 2 ——

Walt Whitman began the Civil War in a deep depression. His career as a poet had burst into the national consciousness in 1855—just six years before the war ignited—with the publication of *Leaves of Grass.* Emerson immediately hailed *Leaves* as the "launch of a great career."

Its opening stanzas were strange, breathtaking.

I celebrate myself, and sing myself
And what I assume you shall assume,
For every atom belonging to me as good belongs to you.

The poem startled readers with an earthy American voice, singing of "the teeming, energetic, inventive masses," and of America's spirit of resilience and nobility. Its pulse was loose, free, and frankly erotic.

> I loaf and invite my soul,
> I lean and loaf at my ease observing a spear of summer grass.
> My tongue, every atom of my blood, formed from this soil, this
>   air,
> Born here of parents born here from parents the same, and their
>   parents the same,
> I, now thirty-seven years old in perfect health begin,
> Hoping to cease not till death.

Leaves of Grass was more than a book of poetry. It was a declaration of the possibilities of American democracy, and the spirit of the individual that democracy sustains. Whitman was a mystic, yes. But he was a new kind of mystic: a mystic of the people.

The times in which Whitman wrote, however, were perilous, and the spirit of Whitman's poetry soon stalled. In the years immediately after the publication of *Leaves of Grass,* the nation spiraled toward civil war, and Whitman himself—even after his initial triumph—was caught in a personal slough of despond. He spent his nights carousing and cruising with his fellow Bohemians in New York's Greenwich Village, and drinking at the notorious Pfaff's beer cellar. He frequented the New York Free Love league in his spare time. He hung out with (and probably slept with) tough young men from the docks and coach houses. All the while, he lived in an attic room in his mother's home, which, though filled with affection, was also saturated with addiction and mental illness.

During the day, Whitman was underemployed variously as a newspaperman and editor. And when not carousing with the handsome coach drivers on the streets of Manhattan, he obsessively edited and revised *Leaves of Grass.* Whitman was stuck. Stuck in his own past. And stuck in a vision of the country that he vastly preferred to the reality he saw around him. His dharma—so potent just a few years before—had dried up under his feet.

—— 3 ——

Dharma callings are more fluid than we would like them to be. These callings can change maddeningly. Just when we settle into a satisfying moment of dharma flowering, the world upends us. Just when we think we have gotten our due reward in a stretch of good dharma road, the car skids off into a ditch.

Katherine, our friend the girls' school dean—not at all unlike Whitman—found herself suddenly shipwrecked after a long stretch of smooth sailing. A once-electrifying vocation had become unaccountably stale, used up, finished. She discovered, like Whitman, that brilliant careers can turn into golden handcuffs. Used up as they may be, they're still hard to leave behind.

Katherine, you will remember, was indeed handcuffed to a worn-out calling. "It's all I can do to drag myself out of the bed in the morning," she told me. "How did this happen? I pictured myself in this job till they carried me out—growing old as the wise elder of the school."

The tortured clinging to an earlier expression of The Gift very often precedes the emergence of some new version. We're aware of the dryness at the center, yes, but this aridity is usually not quite enough to propel us forward. We must first get just a *whiff* of the new. The surprising and intoxicating whiff of a new dharma is quite irresistible.

Katherine, alas, had not yet sniffed out the new. Walt Whitman was about to.

—— 4 ——

Walt Whitman's whiff of his new dharma was characteristically dramatic.

The American Civil War ignited in 1861 with the firing on Fort Sumter in Charleston Harbor. The North was galvanized into action by this event. Soon afterward, Whitman's brother George enthusiastically enlisted in the rapidly gathering Union Army. Whitman and his family were now intimately involved in the young war—through George—and they anxiously scanned the newspaper accounts of battles, paying worried attention to the lists of wounded and dead. In mid-December of

1862, their worst fears were realized. The *New-York Tribune* carried a list of casualties at the bloody battle of Fredericksburg, Virginia, and there appeared on the list one "G. W. Whitmore, Company D."

Could this G. Whitmore really be George Whitman? Walt packed a few clothes, notebooks, and fifty dollars in cash—his household's entire cash reserves—and left for Washington. He was forty-seven years old. His life was about to change.

Walt Whitman spent several desperate days searching for his brother in hospitals all over Washington, D. C. He finally located the very-much-alive—and apparently indestructible—George (who would go on to survive a full twenty Civil War battles). George had been wounded in one cheek, yes, but mildly so, and he had already returned to his regiment. Whitman found him resting comfortably in his tent at the winter encampment.

The search for George had been productive in ways Walt Whitman had not anticipated. It gave him his first exposure to the suffering in Civil War hospitals. And it was during this time that he had his first taste of ministering to wounded and dying soldiers. He found himself drawn to the suffering of these young men, and he began to visit them—to do what he could to salve their torment. In a letter home, he described it:

> I go around from one case to another. I do not see that I do much good, but I cannot leave them. Once in a while some youngster holds on to me convulsively, and I do what I can for him: at any rate, stop with him and sit near him for hours, if he wishes it.

Whitman began to visit the hospitals regularly, drawn by the possibility that he could do some good for "the boys." This was not the result of any high-minded scheme to do good. He simply had allowed events to take their course—a character trait that had always been part of Whitman's genius, and that he wrote about at length in *Song of the Open Road*. Whitman noticed what drew his interest—and then, footloose as he was, he allowed himself to go with it. Today we might call this "going with the flow." The flexibility in Whitman's personality allowed him to attune with surprising dexterity to a wholly new vocation. Careful attunement to dharma will demand that we reinvent ourselves periodically throughout life. Whitman, as it turned out, was a master at self-reinvention.

Whitman's own journals tell the story of one of his first patients: Private John Holmes. Holmes was a twenty-one-year-old soldier from Bridgewater, Massachusetts—a shoemaker by trade. He had seen action at the Battle of Antietam, where he managed to avoid being wounded. But he had nonetheless become victim of the biggest stealth killer of the war: diarrhea. The disease afflicted over half of all Union soldiers. It was a nightmare to suffer through, and for many Civil War soldiers it resulted in a slow, wasting death.

Holmes had suffered a ghastly series of mistreatments at the hands of inept Union medical personnel, until he finally collapsed at Washington's Campbell Hospital, where Whitman found him. Whitman was alarmed by "his glassy eyes, with a look of despair and hopelessness, sunk low in his thin, pallid-brown young face."

"I sat down by him without any fuss," Whitman later wrote in his journal, "talked a little; soon saw that it did him good; led him to talk a little himself; got him somewhat interested; wrote a letter for him to his folks in Massachusetts . . . soothed him down as I saw he was getting a little too much agitated, and tears in his eyes; gave him some small gifts and told him I should come again soon."

Whitman began to see that his mere presence, his tenderness, his attention, had an enormous healing effect. He ministered faithfully to Holmes for weeks and Holmes eventually recovered his health completely and rejoined his unit. But as he left the hospital, John Holmes told Whitman that he believed without question that Whitman had saved his life.

Whitman had found a new calling—a calling for which he didn't even know he was searching. He described it to his brother Jeff: "I cannot give up my Hospitals yet," he wrote. "I never before had my feelings so thoroughly and (so far) permanently absorbed, to the very roots, as by these huge swarms of dear, wounded, sick, dying boys."

As it turned out—and as is so often the case in these matters—his whole life had been a preparation for this dharma. It was a calling that used all of him—itinerant poet, nurse, surrogate father, mother, brother, angel. And being a poet by nature, Whitman soon found precise words for his new calling. He inscribed it on the front of the notebook he would carry throughout the rest of the war: "Walt Whitman, Soldier's Missionary."

— 5 —

Could our friend Katherine find the same flexibility within herself? In recent months, I had seen Katherine's paralysis begin to break up. She had started to sniff around—thinking more actively about what might be next for her. Once she started to really pay attention to her dilemma, she realized that her Plan B—teaching English literature part-time, gardening, and caring for her cats—did not really light her up at all. Much as she might try to spice it up in her own mind, Plan B felt wan, empty, and a little pathetic. It did not have the hallmarks of dharma.

Then, after almost two years of active listening and waiting—her version of Whitman's slough of despond in New York City—Katherine got a whiff of something new, something vividly alive. She called me, excited.

Out of the blue, Katherine had been asked to be the editor of a small and now-struggling journal of nature writing. It had once aimed to be one of the premier journals of great nature writing, and aspired to feature the blossoming Thoreaus and Burroughs of the times. But the journal had fallen on hard times. Katherine had been on their board for six years. (It was one thing that had really lit her up in the previous three years.) And then, quite without warning, an opening: The forty-five-year-old editor had left the journal smack in the middle of the recession. In difficult straits as they were, the journal couldn't pay much. But they needed Katherine's steady and already-trusted hand at the wheel. They had no reason to think she was available. They asked anyway.

Here it was. The intersection of The Gift and The Times. This new work would use Katherine's gifts for writing and editing. Her love of organic gardening. Her devotion to nature. Her concern about the future of the planet. And it cooked them all together into an entirely new stew that Katherine found thrilling. It was small. And it was very, very large.

— 6 —

Walt Whitman passionately adopted the garb of Soldier's Missionary. He began to develop a routine—the essential infrastructure of any profession. He started, as he said, by "fortifying myself with previous rest, the bath, clean clothes, a good meal, and as cheerful an appearance as possible." Before he sallied forth, he prepared a grab bag of treats, including candy, fruit, writing supplies, tobacco, socks, cookies, underwear. He would then set forth to the hospital wards and sessions of "visiting" that might last anywhere from two hours to four or five hours. He embraced his work with everything he had. "Behold," he had written earlier in *Leaves of Grass* (as if foreshadowing his work in the hospitals), "I do not give lectures or a little charity. When I give I give myself."

There is no episode of Whitman's nursing career more moving than his involvement with a young fifer named Erastus Haskell, who contracted typhoid fever while serving with the 141st New York. Whitman describes him as "a silent dark-skinn'd Spanish-looking youth, with large very dark blue eyes . . ."

Doctors had pronounced Haskell's case all but hopeless, and Whitman sat with him as much as he could during his final weeks. "Many nights I sat by in the hospital till far in the night—The lights would be put out—yet I would sit there silently, hours, late, perhaps fanning him—he always liked to have me sit there, but never cared to talk—I shall never forget those nights, it was a curious and solemn scene, the sick and wounded lying around in their cots, just visible in the darkness and this dear young man close at hand lying on what proved to be his death bed—I do not know his past life, but what I do know, and what I saw of him, he was a noble boy."

In a letter to Haskell's parents after the young man's death, Whitman reveals some of the deepest sources of his call:

"I write you this letter, because I would do something at least in his memory—his fate was a hard one, to die so—He is one of the thousands of our unknown American men in the ranks about whom there is no record or fame, no fuss made about their dying so unknown, but I find in them the real precious and royal ones of this land, giving themselves up, aye even their young and precious lives, in their country's cause . . ."

Whitman gave his boys the gift of acknowledging the nobility of their sacrifice. He faced death with them.

— 7 —

By the fall of 1863, Whitman had begun to feel the strain of death and loss. He was increasingly distracted and emotional, and he wrote at length to his mother about his "heart-sickness." Whitman had taken on the suffering of the times. He began to write poetry again as a way of coming to terms with this suffering. Now, his experience in the war spilled forth in a swell of words: newspaper articles, essays, poems.

Whitman would later collect his war poems into a volume entitled *Drum-Taps.* He wanted, he said, "to express in a poem . . . the pending action of this *Time and Land we swim in,* with all their large conflicting fluctuations of despair and hope, the shiftings, masses, and the whirl and deafening din . . . the unprecedented anguish of wounded and suffering."

Through his writing, Whitman attempts to see into the soul of the soldier. He finds their souls to be immortal.

I see behind each mask that wonder a kindred soul,
O the bullet could never kill what you really are, dear friend,
Nor the bayonet stab what you really are;
the Soul! Yourself I see, great as any, good as the best,
Waiting secure and content, which the bullet could never kill,
Nor the bayonet stab O friend.

Whitman gave no indication in his journal that he had studied the Bhagavad Gita. But in his poetry he declared over and over again the very same truth that Krishna taught to Arjuna on the field of Kurukshetra: "Our bodies are known to end, but the embodied self is enduring, indestructible, and immeasurable . . . Weapons do not cut it, fire does not burn it, waters do not wet it . . . it is enduring, all-pervasive, fixed, immovable, and timeless."

Like the ancient Seer, Whitman had seen through the mask of death. He became the witness—the gray-bearded Seer—for his generation, and for the world. He was a witness to the nobility of spirit that emerged in the center of cataclysm, of massacre, of war. Walt Whitman, Soldier's Missionary, became the Krishna of the times—seeing the madness, speaking it, grieving wildly for the loss of precious life and innocence. He took on the task—a devouring task—of understanding the meaning of the war.

By the end of the war, Whitman the poet seemed to be everywhere. He was at the front lines of the battle. He was in the hospital tents. He was there when the Grand Review happened at the end of the war—the great parade in Washington, D.C. that marched out the whole tattered lot of generals and enlisted men and wounded men and congressmen and secretaries of war. Whitman was there—Seer-like—near the platform that held all the dignitaries, and saw and described the actors—President Johnson (Lincoln had been assassinated just weeks before), the generals, the secretary of war. But he would always say that the rank and file were the ones who most drew his love, attention, and admiration.

— 8 —

Katherine's friends were not thrilled with her anticipated reinvention of herself. They had imagined another future for her. They had assumed that she would be joining them for bridge, luncheons, and garden club. They had not imagined her going to work at a faltering magazine, meeting deadlines, carrying what seemed to them a great new burden. They pushed against it.

"It's true," Katherine admitted to me in a moment of doubt. "The job is not perfect." The work, after all, was tedious at times. Crazy hours. The future of the journal was entirely unknown. God knows it would probably always be shaky financially. Why on earth would she trade in a comfortable position in the big brick buildings of the school for an ancient farmhouse whose unpainted outbuildings were crumbling? This was a job for a much younger person.

Her friends were alarmed. "It will use you up, Katherine."

But this carping was enough to push her to the other side of her ambivalence (ambivalence, it turns out, is an unavoidable companion in the search for a new dharma): "Well, what if it does?" she countered. "What else do I have to be used up by? My cats?"

We in twenty-first-century America have strange dreams and fantasies about retirement. We imagine a life of leisure. The Golden Years. But what is this leisure in the service of?

When we reach sixty-two, as Katherine had, we are likely to interpret feelings of exhaustion and boredom as the signal to retire. But couldn't they just as easily be the call to reinvent ourselves? As we age it seems harder and harder to let our authentic dharma reinvent us. We imagine somehow that the risks are greater. We tend to think that leaping off cliffs is for the young. But no. Actually—when better to leap off cliffs? (T. S. Eliot said it: "Old men ought to be explorers.")

The fear of leaping is, of course, the fear of death. It is precisely the fear of being used up. And dharma does use us up, to be sure. But why not be used up giving everything we've got to the world? This is precisely what Krishna teaches Arjuna: You cannot hold on to your life. You don't need to. You are immortal. "Our bodies are known to end, but the embodied self is enduring, indestructible, and immeasurable; therefore, Arjuna, fight the battle!"

The Gift is not for its own sake. It is for the common good. It is for The Times.

—— 9 ——

At the end of the war it became Walt Whitman's self-assigned duty to make sense of its unimaginable suffering—including Lincoln's assassination, which came just days after Lee's surrender to Grant at Appomattox. Right away, Whitman saw the meaning of the assassination—and he saw it in Krishnean terms: "He was assassinated—but the Union is not assassinated . . . The Nation is immortal."

Whitman began to work on an elegy to describe the meaning of the war. He called it, "Retrievements Out of the Night." It was perhaps his greatest poem. It was written for all the bruised and broken young men. The poem was saturated with death:

Come lovely and soothing death,
Undulate round the world, serenely arriving, arriving,
In the day, in the night, to all, to each,
Sooner or later delicate death.

Here were commingled the memories of the dead soldiers and their dead commander—the president. It was a triumph of a poem—written in the thrall of dharma. It was the last great poem of Whitman's career.

Whitman's poetic genius could not be for himself alone. His deeper gifts revealed themselves when put in the service of the times and of the greatest need. Having been put in the service of humanity, his gift was ennobled, transformed. His words helped turn the dark wound of the Civil War into a kind of transcendent light. Whitman had developed an expansive consciousness that saw into the meaning of things. This is, after all, what a poet does. He had infused his poetic spirit into his "missionary" work in the hospitals. He had turned his life into a poem—a work of art—in the most unlikely of places: the Civil War hospital tent.

We see here the themes that will occupy the rest of the book: Selflessness. Sacrifice. Surrender. Not just responsibility to The Gift itself, but responsibility to give it *in the way that is called forth.* Krishna says, "Strive constantly to serve the welfare of the world; by devotion to selfless work one attains the supreme goal of life. Do your work with the welfare of others always in mind."

By the end of the war, Whitman was used up. The photographs of him before and after the war show him stunningly aged and transformed. Through his work in the hospital tents he gave himself away. But he also found himself.

After the war, Whitman experienced a long, slow decline in health. He would never be the same. But he did not count the cost. "There were years in my life—years there in New York—when I wondered if all was not going to the bad with America—the tendency downwards—but the war saved me: what I saw in the war set me up for all time—the days in the hospitals."

The Civil War saved the Union. But it also saved Walt Whitman. It saved him from a life trapped in self. It called forth from him his highest, noblest vision of mankind—and in speaking this vision, he made it so.

Like Thoreau, he had discovered the power of authentic words to change the world.

Dharma is born mysteriously out of the intersection between The Gift and The Times. Dharma is a response to the urgent—though often hidden—need of the moment. Each of us feels some aspect of the world's suffering acutely. It tears at our hearts. Others don't see it or don't care. But we feel it. And we must pay attention. We must act. This little corner of the world is ours to transform. This little corner of the world is ours to save.

PART III

The Second Pillar: "Do It Full Out!"

I was wandering aimlessly through an art gallery in New York City several years ago when I was stopped in my tracks by a stunning Japanese print. It was Katsushika Hokusai's *The Great Wave off Kanagawa*—a stylized print of a mammoth and looming wave framing a distant mountain. I vaguely remembered studying this picture in a college art course. Wasn't there something about the "innovative artistic tension-arc" created by the moving wave in the foreground and the small-but-unmoving presence of the mountain anchoring the distance? Yes, I could see it now. More than that, I could *feel* it. In person—at midlife—the print had an energy and power of which I had been oblivious as a college sophomore.

Even more than the print itself, however, I was captivated by the artist's words about his work—posted on a small ivory card next to the print: "From around the age of six," the artist began, "I had the habit of sketching from life." He continues:

"I became an artist, and from fifty on began producing works that won some reputation, but nothing I did before the age of seventy was worthy of attention. At seventy-three, I began to grasp the structures of birds and beasts, insects and fish, and of the way plants grow. If I go on trying, I will surely understand them still better by the time I am eighty-six, so that by ninety I will have penetrated to their essential nature. At one hundred, I may well have a positively divine understanding of them, while at one-hundred and thirty, forty, or more I will have reached the stage where every dot and every stroke I paint will be alive. May Heaven, that grants long life, give me the chance to prove that this is no lie."

Every dot and stroke I paint will be alive!

Here was a man who was on fire for his work. I wanted to know more: Did he indeed live to be a hundred and forty? What did those later dots and strokes look like?"

I sat down on the bench in front of the print and made some notes. "Katsushika Hokusai. 1760–1849. Japanese printmaker. Leading Japanese expert on Chinese painting. Master of the Ukiyo-e form. Nichiren Buddhist."

Later, at home, I Googled Hokusai. He died at eighty-nine, and sure enough, on his deathbed—still looking to penetrate deeper into his art—he had exclaimed, "If only heaven will give me just another ten years! . . . Just another five more years, then I could become a real painter."

Hokusai was a man who saw his work as a means to "penetrate to the essential nature" of things. And he appears to have succeeded. His work, a hundred and fifty years after his death, could reach right off a gallery wall and grab me in the gut.

More than anything, I was intrigued by the quality of Hokusai's passion for his work. He helped me see that a life devoted to dharma can be a deeply ardent life.

—— 2 ——

In the first part of "the wondrous dialogue," Krishna and Arjuna speak of dharma—its nature, and its role on the path of the fully alive human being. We have spoken so far of what we might call the *discernment phase* of dharma—the process of sniffing out dharma at every turn. Now comes a new phase: Having found your dharma, embrace it fully and passionately. Bring everything you've got to it. *Do it full out!*

"Considering your dharma, you should not vacillate," Krishna instructed Arjuna. The vacillating mind is the split mind. The vacillating mind is the doubting mind—the mind at war with itself. "The ignorant, indecisive and lacking in faith, waste their lives," says Krishna. "They can never be happy in this world or any other." Ouch.

Well, this Hokusai character was a guy who had not dithered on the path, and had clearly not wasted his life. In fact, he doesn't seem to have wasted an instant. An interesting aspect of fulfilled lives is that the people who are living them seem to have learned how to gather their energy, how to focus—how to, as we might say these days, "bring it." Like Hokusai, their lives begin to look like guided missiles.

How exactly do they accomplish this? How do you get from where most of us live—the run-of-the-mill split mind—to the gathered mind of a Hokusai?

Krishna articulates the principle succinctly: Acting in unity with your purpose *itself* creates unification. Actions that consciously support dharma have the power to begin to gather our energy. These outward actions, step-by-step, shape us inwardly. Find your dharma and do it. And in the process of *doing* it, energy begins to gather itself into a laser beam of effectiveness.

Krishna quickly adds: Do not worry about the outcome. Success or failure are not your concern. It is better to fail at your own dharma than to succeed at the dharma of another. Your task is only to bring as much life force as you can muster to the execution of your dharma. In this spirit, Chinese Master Guan Yin Tzu wrote: "Don't waste time calculating your chances of success and failure. Just fix your aim and begin."

Krishna now begins the task of teaching Arjuna the Doctrine of Unified Action, which explicitly lays out the case for focus. The Doctrine of Unified Action is a pillar of the yoga tradition. The word yoga, in all its various iterations, always and everywhere means "to yoke." In the case of the yoga of action, it means to yoke all of one's being to dharma. To bring every action into alignment with your highest purpose. To bring everything you've got to the task.

American writer Annie Dillard stumbled onto this principle early on in her writing career. She declares it in her book *The Writing Life*. "One of the few things I know about writing is this: Spend it all, shoot it, play it, lose it, all, right away, every time. Do not hoard what seems good for a later place in the book, or for another book; give it, give it all, give it now. The impulse to save something good for a better place later is the signal to spend it now. Something more will arise for later, something better. These things fill from behind, from beneath, like well water. The impulse to keep to yourself what you have learned is not only shameful, it is destructive. Anything you do not give freely and abundantly becomes lost to you."

Give freely and abundantly! Abundance is a central aspect of this principle. When you commit fully to the task at hand, the abundance of your commitment itself has magic in it. It draws your energies together. It calls up energies you didn't know you had. As some have said, under these conditions the universe comes to your aid.

Naturally, there is an obstacle to all this wonderment. Alas, it turns out that the process of unification requires saying "no" to actions that do not support dharma—saying "no" to detours, and to side channels of all kinds, even to some pretty terrific side channels. It requires snipping off all manner of "other options." The root of the word "decide" means, literally, "to cut off." To decide *for* something means at times to decide *against* something else.

This is, of course, why those infernal crossroads are so difficult. Cutting off options is hard work. And it is risky. But the alternative is even riskier. Those who cannot commit, those who cannot say "no," are doomed to everlasting conflict. They may sit for a lifetime at the crossroads, dithering. Krishna nails this principle: "Those who follow this path, resolving deep within themselves to see Me alone, attain singleness of purpose. For those who lack resolution, the decisions of life are many-branched and endless." Many-branched and endless. How well we know.

Because this principle is so important, and because Arjuna is so very likely to lose his tenuous grasp on it, Krishna reminds him over and over again throughout their dialogue. "The disunited mind is far from wise," he nudges. The mind "must overcome the confusion of duality."

If we have been paying the slightest attention to decades of self-help literature, we will not have failed to have heard this same cry. I particularly like American writer Elbert Hubbard's hefty jab for unification: "The difference in men does not lie in the size of their hands, nor in the perfection of their bodies, but in this one sublime ability of concentration: to throw the weight in one blow, to live eternity in an hour."

We derive the greatest pleasure and fulfillment when all our faculties are drawn together into our life's work. In this state of absorption, we experience extraordinary satisfaction. We human beings are attracted to the experience of *intense involvement*. The outcome of this involvement, says Hokusai, is sublime. "By ninety I will have penetrated to their essential nature." Hokusai's lesson, finally, is that a life of passion for dharma is a fulfilled life.

In Part III, then, we will explore the Second Pillar of Dharma, "Do It Full Out!" And we'll look at three principles of the Doctrine of Unified Action.

1. Find out who you are and do it on purpose.
2. Unify!
3. Practice deliberately.

In Chapter Five, we will examine the early life of the American poet Robert Frost, looking closely at the way he made decisions in support of dharma. In Chapter Six, we will examine the surprising life of Susan B. Anthony, and the many ways in which she systematically unified her energy, becoming, finally, an authentic force of nature. And in Chapter Seven, we will look at one of the world's greatest landscape painters, the nineteenth-century French master Camille Corot, and examine closely our growing understanding of the concept of "deliberate practice" and its intriguing relationship to dharma. Along the way, we'll look, too, at two ordinary lives—those of my friends Ethan and Lonny—and the ways in which they do or do not manage to grasp the full import of unified action.

FIVE

Robert Frost: Find Out Who You Are and Do It on Purpose

At eighteen years of age I arrived as a first-year student at Amherst College, (a small liberal arts college in western Massachusetts), fresh-plucked from the farm in Ohio. I knew oh-so-little about life. And almost nothing about New England, into whose throbbing heart I had just been transplanted. I knew nothing about her saints and poets and mystics. I knew nothing, even, about one of her chief priests: the poet Robert Frost.

This would soon change. I discovered that the mammoth fact of Robert Frost could simply not be avoided—especially at Amherst College. Frost himself had died a few years before I arrived, and this had given wings to the legend. His name was everywhere, and the college reveled in its association with him. The new Robert Frost Library had just been completed, with its rough-hewn granite foundation, and its more delicate brick and glass stories above. The poet, everyone said, "would have approved."

If that were not enough, several of my new friends in college had committed some portion of Frost's canon to memory, and were apt to recite Frost's poems at the least provocation. Imagine with me, if you will, one such new friend whom I will call Ethan—who will represent the spirit of many of my new friends who had fallen in love with, and could freely recite, Robert Frost. Occasionally these recitations were haunting—as when Ethan and I and two other friends huddled around a campfire on a late October camping trip to Vermont. We had just spent the day hiking through woods blazing with fall color, and I was on fire with the flinty smell and feel of New England. To complete the mood, Ethan treated us to a mesmerizing recitation of "The Road Not Taken"— astonishingly enough, my first hearing of Robert Frost's most ubiquitous poem. I will never forget it. The sweet-acrid smell of the woods, the glow-in-the-dark faces of my new friends around the fire, the intentionally slow, incantatory tone of Ethan's voice.

> Two roads diverged in a yellow wood,
> And sorry I could not travel both
> And be one traveler, long I stood
> And looked down one as far as I could
> To where it bent in the undergrowth;
>
> Then took the other, as just as fair,
> And having perhaps the better claim,
> Because it was grassy and wanted wear;
> Though as for that the passing there
> Had worn them really about the same,
>
> And both that morning equally lay
> In leaves no step had trodden black.
> Oh, I kept the first for another day!
> Yet knowing how way leads on to way,
> I doubted if I should ever come back.
>
> I shall be telling this with a sigh
> Somewhere ages and ages hence:
> Two roads diverged in a wood, and I—
> I took the one less traveled by,
> And that has made all the difference.

When he finished there was silence, save for the crackling of the fire. And into the silence, several minutes later, Ethan "said" the poem again. (Frost famously "said" his poems, rather than "recited" them.)

I was an eighteen-year-old, and had just made the first major decision of my life: the choice of a college. Would it be Amherst, or the College of Wooster, in Ohio, or Hamilton College, in New York? Of course, I did not have the word "dharma" in my vocabulary then. But the college choice had been the biggest dharma decision of my life thus far. The poem Ethan recited that magical night—which is about what we do at crossroads—was full of hidden meaning and import for me. I secretly believed this very camping trip proved that I had chosen well. Look where I was. And who I was with: exotic new friends who recited poetry in the woods at night. Look what a turn my life had taken out of the mundanity (as I thought) of Ohio. My decision was the right one. And I was experiencing the power of choice. *Observe,* I thought: I had already taken the road less traveled.

Frost haunted me. At first entirely through Ethan. But the poet slowly became my own. From my first hearing of Frost's words, I felt some strange kinship with him, as if his was a voice I had known somewhere long, long ago, and was just rediscovering. He evoked in me a kind of nostalgia for a past that seemed to have faded into a near dream.

Strangely, Frost describes his own process of *making poetry* in a very similar fashion—as a kind of homecoming to a lost part of himself. "For me," he says, "the initial delight is in the surprise of remembering something I didn't know I knew." In a new poem, he wrote, he "meets himself coming home."

By the time I returned to Ohio for Christmas vacation, I had already committed my first Frost poem to memory. I repeated it to myself over and over again as I walked the snow-swept fields of my boyhood town, as if introducing my past to my future. I loved the feel of the words in my mouth:

Some say the world will end in fire,
Some say in ice.
From what I've tasted of desire
I hold with those who favor fire.
But if I had to perish twice,
I think I know enough of hate

To say that for destruction ice
Is also great
And would suffice.

Some say the world will end in fire. Oh, the sound of it! Before I left for Ohio, I "said" this poem once in Ethan's presence, rattling it off with poorly disguised pride while on a hike across the Holyoke Range. He smiled but said nothing.

—— 2 ——

Frost, of course, became the most lauded American poet of his century—winning no less than four Pulitzer Prizes (a record) and single-handedly remaking American poetry.

His life is, then, naturally, a treasure trove of stories about dharma. But to my mind, the most interesting story is the series of courageous early choices Frost made in support of his dharma. When one examines Frost's life closely, it becomes clear that this man became more and more himself through a *series of small decisions that aligned him with his voice.* He had a gift, of course. But his power came into focus through his *commitment to this gift,* and through a series of decisive actions taken in support of it. Each one of these acts was, for him, like jumping off a cliff. He jumped not entirely blind—but not entirely seeing, either. And each of Frost's leaps ignited more of his power. In retrospect, it is clear that each one of Frost's difficult decisions helped create the perfect conditions for the full flowering of his genius. He chose relentlessly over and over again—in small ways and in large—*for his dharma.* His remarkable career was the fruit of these decisions.

Frost's early years were spent finding out who he was. But his later years were spent increasingly *being who he was on purpose.* As he himself said, the story of his life is the story of someone becoming more and more himself. He later wrote:

They would not find me changed from him they knew—
Only more sure of all I thought was true.

— 3 —

From early on, Robert Frost had an ear for "voice"—for the good story, the compelling colloquialism, the rough-hewn sound of local speech. Very often, he discovered the power of words—and their flinty patterns— while he was at work. Even as a boy, Frost loved physical work. "I liked to try myself out in a job," he once recalled, "helping a man load a wagon, pile firewood, rake or hoe. It was all odd jobs in those days. I liked working with characters, listening to them, their stories, the way they had to tell a story—the country was full of characters."

Young Robbie loved hearing his mother read to him at night. He felt soothed by her voice. And his imagination was alive with the stories she read: Walter Scott's *Tales of a Grandfather;* traditional ballads; Scottish tales. Also poetry: Ossian, Poe, Wordsworth, Longfellow, and Bryant.

Frost's life developed an interesting rhythm: working on a farm during the day—haying, using a pitchfork, learning how to use a scythe. And studying the classics at night. He studied poetry. He read the Latin poets. He began to tinker with writing small poems, especially as a way of integrating moments of powerful feeling.

Frost himself told and retold the story of writing his first poem. The poem, later published by *The Independent,* was titled, "My Butterfly." He was just twenty years old. "I wrote it all in one go in the kitchen of our house on Tremont Street," Frost said. "I locked the door and all the time I was working, Jeanie my sister tried to batter it down and get in." And as he wrote that first poem, Frost recalls, he had a profound sense that "something was happening. It was like cutting along a nerve."

I have often heard artists describe this "cutting along a nerve." Sculptor Anne Truitt said, "The most demanding part of living a lifetime as an artist is the strict discipline of forcing oneself to work steadfastly along the nerve of one's own most intimate sensitivity." Frost found the experience exhilarating.

"My Butterfly" was Frost's first published poem. When *The Independent* editor William Hayes Ward saw it, he recognized the genius there. Ward later questioned Frost: Who are you? Where did you come from? What was your education? Frost had to admit to Ward that he did not have a college education at all. He declared that it was his love for poetry—and his ambition to write *great* poetry—that had compelled his self-training. "To love poetry is to study it," he said to Ward. (Frost became one of America's greatest autodidacts.)

By the age of twenty, Frost had fallen in love with words, and had decided that he would be a poet—though he did not know how this would come to be. He set himself very intentionally on a training program to study the great poets. "Specifically speaking," he said to Ward, "the few rules I know in this art are my own afterthoughts, or else directly formulated from the masterpieces I reread."

—— 4 ——

My friend Ethan's early life resembled Frost's in surprising ways. His parents owned a dairy farm in Vermont, and he grew up with the same earthbound rhythms that Frost loved so much. He often said to me, "Frost is telling me my own life."

Ethan was a tall, intense young man, with dark eyes and thick, tightly curled chestnut hair. He walked on the earth with an unmistakable lope, like a cougar stalking its prey. I could always spot Ethan's distinctive walk across the busy expanse of the Amherst quads.

I had met Ethan on our very first day at college—both of us sitting alone and forlorn at the top of what is called "Memorial Hill," looking out over the distant Mount Holyoke Range and wondering how the heck we'd gotten ourselves in so far over our heads. We were both socially out of our element: he a farm boy from rural Vermont, me a rube from the cornfields of Ohio. We recognized in each other a kindred spirit. And over the course of those first few months of struggle we became inseparable.

Ethan was driven to succeed. I didn't even know what "driven" was then. I did not have that quality—nor did anyone in my family. But I knew that Ethan was unlike anyone I had ever met. He was good at whatever he put his hand to: soccer, lacrosse, baseball—a golden boy on the playing fields. Later, when I met his lovely and soft-spoken parents, I wondered where his intensity came from. Not from them. They were thrilled to have a son in college at all. Stardom was not required of him. He'd already succeeded in their eyes.

In addition to sports, Ethan was in love with poetry. He knew from that first day on Memorial Hill that he wanted to be an English major. Ethan taught me how to read poetry in late-night sessions sprawled out in the first-floor lounge of our dorm. Sometimes we spent nights reading poetry together and critiquing it. We went for long hikes on the Holyoke Range. Ethan and I were the same age, almost exactly, but he seemed to me more like an older brother. He was much wiser than I—or so I thought then.

Ethan introduced me to Thoreau, and we cut a day of classes in the spring to visit Walden Pond, which we approached like a trip to a great shrine. He was particularly in love with Thoreau's insights about "the wild," because he felt a wildness in himself that he did not understand. Even in freshman year, Ethan was thinking about becoming a writer. He spent some of his spare time working on short stories and poems, and talked to me about a novel he had cooking away in his head. He wanted to know everything about writing.

Part of Ethan's wildness came out on the playing fields. He was intensely competitive. I didn't understand this side of him. Ethan would become moody around game time and afterward. He was exuberant if he won, devastated if he lost—and highly critical of his performance in either case. His moods sometimes scared me. He said his mother called them "spells." In fact, his mother actually took me aside once and asked me if Ethan had been having "spells." Of course I had no idea that this wildness in him would later turn in on itself—as it did on Frost, who was dogged by depression throughout his life.

— 5 —

With the publication of "My Butterfly," Frost had gone public with his poetry. And he was getting a great deal of positive response. After reading "Butterfly," a friend of Ward's offered to be young Frost's literary advisor. This "advisor" then proceeded to give the young Robert Frost one of the most misguided pieces of counsel ever given to a great poet. He suggested that Frost try for "a more elevated tone." His poetry was "too close to the speaking voice," he declared.

Frost was incensed. The speaking voice was his direct line into truth—into the heart of poetry itself. He wanted, in fact, to write poetry that would mine *precisely* this rich ore of human speech. *Too close to the speaking voice?* It was misguided advice, yes, but the confrontation itself had a silver lining. It became the opportunity for Frost himself to understand exactly what he was doing. It was the moment when he made explicit the connection between the *sounds of poetry* and the *sounds of ordinary speech.* This discovery was one of the central epiphanies of Frost's life, and he would later describe it as a crossroads experience.

"Perhaps," wrote Frost later, "when that preacher friend of Ward's looked me up shortly after my first poem appeared in *The Independent* and talked to me about it, something providential was happening to me. I'm sure the old gentleman didn't have the slightest idea he was having any effect on a very stubborn youngster who thought he knew what he knew. But something he said actually changed the whole course of my writing. It all became purposeful."

I once heard country-and-western singer Dolly Parton declare a stunning bit of truth: "Find out who you are," she said, "and then do it on purpose." This homespun proverb is a gloss on Robert Frost's life. *Find out who you are and do it on purpose.*

For the first time, Frost knew what he was after. And he began to do it on purpose. He started calling his poems "talk songs." He discovered that the rhythm of his most authentic poetic voice came very close to prose, but "is lifted just enough so that it stays inside the boundary lines of verse." Frost came to call his voice the "sound of sense."

He exulted in this discovery. "The sound of sense!" he exclaimed. "It is the . . . vitality of our speech. It is pure sound—pure form. One who concerns himself with it more than the subject is an artist."

The sound of sense! This is precisely what I had first loved in Frost's poetry. *Some say the world will end in fire, some say in ice.* I loved the way the words *felt* in my mouth. He had captured the sounds of real life, and distilled out of them their very music. This is what Ethan meant when he said that "Frost was speaking my New England life to me."

Frost discovered that his vocation was to artfully bring the sounds of everyday speech into poetry. He wanted to catch the humanness of speech in his poetic net. He became fascinated with the tension between the classical forms of poetry and the vernacular performance of speech.

Where do the stresses normally fall in speech? He began to experiment with pulling the speech slightly toward the form, and the form slightly toward the speech.

Now Frost was "onto his bone," as Thoreau would say. He knew that this was a task big enough for a lifetime. He knew that he would be chewing on it for the rest of his career. *Bury it, circle 'round it, unearth it, bury it again!*

—— 6 ——

When I arrived back at Amherst after a junior year in South America, something in Ethan had changed. He had abruptly taken up a premed course of study (in preparation for a medical career), and had unaccountably ditched his previous major in English literature. What the hell? How and when did this happen?

Ethan didn't want to talk with me about it. "You were in South America," he complained. "How was I going to talk with you?"

"You didn't think about maybe writing me a letter?" I retorted, hurt.

Ethan *couldn't* explain it to me. I saw later that he couldn't even explain it to himself. He was articulate about absolutely everything else. Why not about this? This need to become a doctor seemed to emerge from some other part of his personality. Perhaps it was related to what happened to him on the playing fields? That competitive part of his spirit—that wildness that I never really understood?

That fall, Ethan and I went on a four-day hiking trip to Vermont. We stayed for a night at his family's farm. Ethan was more remote on this trip than he had been before. His mind seemed to be elsewhere. Had something happened while I was away? He denied that it had. We sat up late into the night staring into the fire.

In the middle of the night, Ethan woke me up. He was sitting on the side of my bed, sobbing. He tried to talk, but couldn't. "I just can't, can't . . . ," he would begin, and then the sobbing would erupt from deep in his gut. Finally it ebbed.

We sat by the window and talked for most of the rest of the night. We took a walk around the farm as the sun was coming up over the yellowing Vermont woods. He felt split, he said. Split right down the middle.

He talked of his love of English, his desire to write poetry, to write prose. To live the life of a writer.

"But it's an impoverished life, Steve. My family, my parents, my sister. I can't let them down. I have to take care of them and I can't take care of them properly if I go down this ruinous course. I cannot do this to them."

Ethan had worked it all out in his mind while I was away. He would become a doctor. He would make plenty of money, and lift his family out of the relative poverty in which they lived. He could help his little sister go to college.

The full story began to spill out: While I was away, Ethan discovered that his father had mortgaged the farm in order to send him to college. As a result of the bumpy economy, the farm was now in serious financial peril—the same farm that had been in the family for four generations. That piece of land was all that was standing between Ethan's family and desolation. They could lose it—because of him.

Ethan and I didn't have the word dharma then. But we did have the word "duty." Close enough. As Ethan saw it, he had a duty. I understood this. It felt like a noble act, and seemed to involve a kind of self-sacrifice I could not even imagine making. We rationalized this together: Medicine would give him an outlet for his brilliant mind, his competitive spirit. And he could write on the weekends, or in the early mornings.

—— 7 ——

By his late twenties, Frost was perfectly aware of his genius, of his life-work, and of the task ahead of him. But he also knew that the systematic cultivation of poetic genius is a high-wire act of human endeavor. He had already announced to his grandfather—who was pushing him to relinquish poetry as a career—that it would take him twenty years to come into his full power as a poet. Frost understood that the poet's chief job is to *create the right conditions for the blossoming of The Gift*. He understood that he needed a chrysalis—a quiet, contemplative life—with plenty of leisure for writing, reading, thinking, contemplating. He intuited that he needed a life set close to nature—nature, which had always been his muse. Frost was intuitively aware of an important principle: In the cultivation of dharma, there is nothing more important than understanding what conditions are needed, and relentlessly creating them.

Frost next made one of the most pivotal decisions of his life: He decided to become a farmer. He bought a farm in Derry, New Hampshire. To his family and friends this seemed a surprising move. But it turned out to be a brilliant one.

Jay Parini, one of Frost's most important biographers, describes the farm that would be Frost's poetic chrysalis: "From all sides of the house the view was appealing. Beyond a rolling hayfield to the east, one saw a large woodlot, composed mostly of maple, oak, and beech. On the south side a stand of alders concealed a west-running brook fed by a pasture spring. A cranberry bog lay nearby. Patches of raspberries and blackberries grew beside the barn, where a sizable vegetable garden could also be found, its contents ready for harvest. There was plenty of space where one might build chicken coops on the north side, beyond the barn."

This would be Frost's laboratory. He would spend the next decade quietly raising poultry in Derry, surrounding himself with the sources of his inspiration by day, and writing poetry in the kitchen every night while the rest of the family slept. "This was a time," said Frost later, "when my eyes and ears were open, very open."

Those who did not understand the genius of Frost's choice to raise poultry found him an inept farmer. Much has been made, too, by Frost biographers of his reputed "laziness." This shows a stunning lack of understanding of Frost's choice. As Robert Penn Warren has observed, "It was a necessary laziness. It was the way his mind, his imagination, worked; he needed all that time, the spaciousness, the ease of getting from day to day. Poems could root in those spaces. In his case, they did."

Frost's gift burst quietly forth during his eleven years in Derry. It was the most sustained period of creativity and generativity in his long life. From the farm he would take many treasures: a close connection with the earth, with the touch and feel and smell of nature, and with the conversation of the plainspoken men and women who surrounded him in an agricultural life. He would draw on this material for the rest of his career.

"It all started in Derry," Frost said. "The whole thing." He had—at some considerable risk—created precisely the right conditions for his dharma. He had taken a risk: He had trusted The Gift.

—— 8 ——

Two years after we graduated from Amherst, I visited Ethan in Boston. He was at the end of his second year of medical school—living in a little apartment near the campus, with his new wife, Betts. I had not met Betts until the wedding—a grand affair that took place at the Ritz-Carlton Hotel in Boston. She was blonde, well-spoken, elegant in every way. And with a toughness that matched Ethan's. I liked her instantly. I thought it was probably a good match in many ways, because she could stand up to Ethan's wildness. But I soon discovered that she didn't like me. She was anxious that Ethan's literary friend would pull him away from his determination to become a great doctor.

Ethan and I had a wonderful visit, though. He talked excitedly about medicine, and he and I looked together into the future as we had so often at Amherst. I could see him making the best of his situation. But we were both nostalgic for college times. He now talked about his love of poetry as naïve, and though he appreciated that aspect of himself, he thought it was best left behind in favor of "really growing up." I swallowed hard at this. Really?

Over the next decade, I watched as Ethan's medical career unfolded brilliantly. Within five years or so he had already begun to make a name for himself in New York, where he had settled after his residency.

Medicine was for Ethan rather akin to the playing fields of college. I could see the competitive, aggressive streak in him coming forward. When I visited Betts and him in their new duplex in Manhattan, I could see a burgeoning concern for money and status. She talked excitedly about her seven-series BMW, their membership in a posh club. She was a shameless name-dropper. I looked at Ethan. Not a trace of embarrassment.

Meanwhile, I had begun to establish myself in Boston. I went to graduate school. I found a partner and I settled down. We bought a house. Ethan and I slowly drifted apart—into very different worlds. I observed to myself from time to time: It is interesting to see the effects of choices as they play themselves out over the long trajectory of life.

— 9 —

Frost's decision to buy the farm in Derry was one of a series of decisions that moved him closer to a full commitment to poetry. The farm was a deeper step in, and he would draw on its inspiration for the rest of his life. But there were more steps to come.

If you bring forth what is within you, it will save you. Frost knew that his calling was going to require more of him. He had not yet fully committed his life to poetry. He was still farming. But too, during the Derry years he had become seriously involved in teaching. He had, at Derry, a busy, complex, and full life.

As Frost brought forth more and more of what was within him, he felt increasingly split. Was he a farmer? A teacher? A poet? He felt a crossroads coming. He knew that if he was going to bring forth what was deepest within him, he would have to commit to it completely. He would have to "try himself," as he said.

At the end of the decade at Derry, now a fully formed poet in command of his voice, he had one more step to take. He would have to take the leap. He would have to declare himself a poet—both to the world and to himself. He would have to explicitly *commit his life to poetry*—to give everything he had.

"No man can know what power he can rightly call his own unless he presses a little," he wrote. It was time to press.

— 10 —

Frost and his wife Elinor would now make a stunning choice. They would sell the farm and move to England, where Robert could devote himself *entirely* to his poetry. This was not an easy choice. In retrospect, of course, it looks obvious. But in the moment, it was not obvious at all. It was a leap off a cliff.

Frost was aware that these kinds of choices meant cutting off other options. He named his great poem "The Road Not Taken," precisely because of his awareness of the possibilities *lost* when one chooses. Frost was properly fascinated with the process of choice. If one looks closely at "The Road Not Taken," one discovers the many ambiguities written there about choice. The "two roads" are, after all, not that very different. "Both that morning equally lay in leaves no step had trodden black," he writes. The signs were vague, indistinct. How to choose?

What Frost makes clear in his poem is that *the act of choosing* is the most important thing. The act of moving forward is what matters. He might have chosen either teaching or poetry. But he had to choose one or the other. He looked long down each path. He understood the loss involved—the cutting off of possibilities. He saw clearly that options once discarded are usually gone forever. Way leads on to way.

But Krishsna writes: *Concerning one's dharma, one should not vacillate!*

Frost was now determined to give himself fully to poetry—to live, as he said, "a life that followed poetically." What followed was an explosion of creativity. Having made his decision, Frost was increasingly on fire with poetry. He would publish his first two books in England—to considerable acclaim—and would return to America several years later a famous poet.

Thoreau, of course, had had an almost identical experience. As soon as he made a commitment to his authentic voice, as soon as he moved back to his *axis mundi,* to Concord, to his immovable spot, his voice gained an energy, a clarity, and a power that it had never had. The choice itself had unleashed something altogether new. *Actions taken in support of dharma change the self. The act of commitment itself calls forth an unseen dharma power.*

This very principle was often invoked by the German philosopher Goethe, and it was vividly articulated by the English explorer W. A. Murray when he was writing about his own dharma choices—particularly his decision to undertake an expedition to the summit of Mount Everest. He wrote: "Until one is committed there is hesitancy, the chance to draw back, always ineffectiveness."

Murray continues: "Concerning all acts of initiative, and creation, there is one elementary truth, the ignorance of which kills countless ideas and splendid plans: That the moment one definitely commits oneself then Providence moves too. All sorts of things occur to help one that would never otherwise have occurred. A whole stream of events issues from the decision, raising in one's favor all manner of unforeseen incidents and meetings and material assistance, which no man could have dreamt would come his way. I have learned a deep respect for one of Goethe's concepts: 'Whatever you can do, or dream you can do, Begin it. Boldness has genius, power, and magic in it.' "

Boldness has magic in it. Frost understood this principle. He saw that his decision to take the leap, to move to England, to fully commit to poetry, had given birth to some entirely new energy and creativity in himself. Most likely everyone who has committed himself to dharma has independently discovered this same phenomenon.

— 11 —

Several years ago, I was in New York raising money for our Institute. Thomas, one of my board members, a prominent doctor, asked me to join him briefly at a cocktail party before we headed off for a business dinner. I arrived at a stunning penthouse on the Upper East Side of Manhattan. And I was completely unaware, until I saw the sign on the door, that I had just arrived at the New York apartment of my long-absent friend Ethan. I could barely breathe as we entered the foyer.

I hadn't seen Ethan in fifteen years. But there he was. I saw him immediately from across the room, and he looked remarkably the same as he had the last time I'd seen him. Handsome. Tanned. And holding forth loudly to a group of suited men and women. He seemed angry. I quickly had the sinking feeling that something was off here. Was Ethan drunk? He was publicly berating one of the younger men in the group, who turned out to be one of his young associates. Everyone was embarrassed. Where was Betts, I wondered? What in the world was going on?

Ethan didn't recognize me at first. Fifteen years had made a difference in my appearance. I realized that if I did not introduce myself, Ethan would never know I was there. I wondered for a moment if I wanted to "meet" him again, especially under these awkward circumstances.

I did introduce myself. Ethan was stiff in response, and made an awkward joke to the group. I was stunned. There was no warmth. He quickly made a comment about getting together, but I doubted that I would hear from him.

I was shaking—with trauma or with anger, I don't know which. Thomas took me aside and told me the story: Ethan had not practiced medicine for many years—relying instead on the considerable fortune that Betts had inherited from her father, and dedicating his life to golf and to making the rounds of New York society. Now the couple was involved in a very public and very nasty divorce. But all of that aside, confessed Thomas, Ethan had long ago become a boor—a trait apparently fueled by too much alcohol. And we had caught him well into his cups that night.

As I said good-bye to Ethan, I was barely breathing. Just for a moment, he seemed to crack. Did I see some trace of embarrassment? There was something in his eyes, certainly.

I felt as though I had just been part of a scene from a bad movie. How ever had Ethan ended up like this? My board member friend and I went out for a couple of drinks, and then on to dinner. We talked late into the night, examining the trajectory of our lives. I told him of the Ethan I had known in college. Of the decisions I had been witness to—decisions that in retrospect may have led Ethan away from his authentic calling.

A life is built on a series of small course corrections—small choices that add up to something mammoth. What string of fateful decisions had landed Ethan so very far from home?

— 12 —

Robert Frost's archetypal poems are often about a journey: A lone wanderer is lost in a swamp, untethered from his inner moorings. How shall he decide which direction to go? How will he find his way out of the swamp? A hiker is caught on the side of a mountain in a storm. Should he continue on to the summit or turn back? In these poetic treks through the inner wilderness, almost every moment is a crossroads. The hiker must pay close attention—must listen, must look, must feel. The choices made at each crossroads are cumulative—and irreversible.

Looking back at his life with the perspective of old age, Robert Frost saw with some satisfaction the series of decisions that led to his fulfillment as a poet. *I shall be telling this with a sigh somewhere ages and ages hence.* He saw clearly how each decision marked a deeper commitment of his time, energy, and life force to the project of his poetry. With each step he cut off other options. Where did he find the courage?

Frost's genius—like Thoreau's, like Goodall's, like Whitman's—was at least in part his willingness to create the right conditions for his dharma to issue forth. His dharma required a farm—and so he bought one. His dharma required him to give up teaching—and so he relinquished it. His dharma required a period of intense work in England—and so he went.

Like Frost's, our job is to make choices that create the right conditions for dharma to flourish. The Gift is indestructible. It is a seed. We are not required to be God. We are not required to create the seed. Only to plant it wisely and well.

SIX

Susan B. Anthony: Unify!

In the last chapter we examined the ways in which life choices give birth to dharma. We saw how Robert Frost—through the cumulative effect of small but critical life decisions—became the midwife of his own dharma. Now we observe a bold progression: Having first named and claimed our dharma, we next begin *to systematically organize all of our life's energies around our calling.* The dharma gradually becomes a point of radiance that focuses and unites our life force. Our lives begin to move into orbit around our vocation.

The unification of life's energies around dharma is a central pillar of Krishna's teaching to Arjuna. Krishna teaches that one must attain "singleness of purpose." "For those who lack resolution, the decisions of life are many-branched and endless," he exhorts Arjuna (as you will recall). For the mind that is "disunited," he says, life is full of suffering. Indeed, under such conditions of disunity, it becomes impossible to bring forth dharma at all. Rather, says Krishna, "The wise [must] unify their consciousness." In this chapter we will explore the stunning possibilities of the unified mind.

Certain components of this "unified mind" have been exhaustively commented upon in the literature of optimal living. Many teachers have chosen to use the word "focus"—as I have at times in this book—and have noted that this selfsame focus is a universal quality of successful lives. Steven Covey, author of *The Seven Habits of Highly Successful Peo-*

ple, cites focus as an essential condition of life mastery. "Winners focus," says author Sydney Harris, "losers spray."

But the Bhagavad Gita gives us a new piece of this puzzle. Not just any old focus will do. Life's energies are most fruitfully focused around *dharma.* Krishna is concerned with the unification of thoughts, words, and actions in alignment with *our soul's highest calling.*

To organize life's energies around anything less sublime than our true nature is to still be split—separated from Self. No matter how much focus we may bring to any task, if the task is not our real vocation we will still be haunted by the suffering of doubt, and the internal agony of division. (There it is again: We cannot be anyone we want to be.)

If you have had the experience of Unity of Action, even briefly, you'll know what I'm talking about. Perhaps once in your life, for just a few months, or weeks, or days, you knew what you were really about. You knew what you had to do, and you did it with passion—with everything you had. You discovered the magic of aim! Somehow, you managed to organize everything in your life to support your aim. Your life, just briefly, was a guided missile of dharma. Have you had this experience?

I once had an experience of this "unified mind" off and on over the course of about four years. It was the most exhilarating four years of my life. I was writing my first book. The Kripalu Center had gone into breakdown. We had fired our spiritual director in the midst of the seemingly inevitable scandal, and everything fell apart around us. The halls were empty of guests. The immense brick building on the hill was a ghost town. Overnight, I had acquired the leisure of Robert Frost on his Derry farm. And I knew what I had to do. I had to write.

For four years, after this surprising bolt of certitude, my life was organized around writing. I rented a quiet office off campus so that I wouldn't be distracted. There was no phone in the office. No Internet on the computer. I did my best to sleep well, to wake early, and to eat simply so that my head would be clear each morning when I arrived at the office. Every morning, from 8 to 11:30, I wrote.

The focus was exhilarating. For the first time in my life, everything was lined up around a clear dharma assignment. And I discovered a secret: *Bringing forth what is within you is mostly about creating the right conditions.* These conditions themselves give birth to dharma. The farmer tills the soil, waters, fertilizes, and weeds. The plant, mystically, does its own growing. I had a motto: Suit up and show up. That's all I had to do! Show up every morning in the best possible shape for writing. I was an Olympic athlete in training. I had for once in my life become that guy who jumps out of bed in the morning.

Once you've had a taste of Unity in Action, nothing else seems quite like living fully.

If you look closely, you will see that the process of "unification of action" is exemplified in every life we have looked at so far. It is there in Goodall, Thoreau, Whitman, Frost. But we are going to add a new life here that exemplifies it in stunning fashion. This is the surprising life of Susan B. Anthony. Here is a story of the way in which a unified life changes not only the person living it, but the whole world.

— 2 —

No great character in American history has been more ill-served by stereotyping, lame biographies, and stuffy hagiography than Susan B. Anthony, the great nineteenth-century champion of women's rights. This magnificent woman is generally seen as a wizened, tight-lipped old do-gooder who probably hated men, sex, and most of the normal pleasures of life. Nothing could be further from the truth. Anthony was a charming, eloquent, and commanding woman who routinely faced down halls of boorish, rude, and obstinate men—and who almost single-handedly created the national strategy that led to the enfranchisement of women. She loved passionately, she worked single-mindedly, and she savored the pleasures of life.

At her funeral in 1906, during a raging blizzard in upstate New York, over 10,000 mourners passed by her flag-draped coffin to pay their respects. Telegrams came in from great world leaders. She was pronounced "the American Moses" from pulpits around the country. Newspapers called her "the American Joan of Arc."

How do we account for such a life? Anthony began life as a shy Quaker girl—given to melancholy, "fragility," and extreme self-doubt. She spent her early years under the care of a clinically depressed mother. As a child, Susan practiced "piety" and "humility"—being seen but not heard, as befitted the prevailing view of the well-brought-up American girl. She was clearly shy. She was probably depressed. How, then, did she become transformed into one of the most powerful women in American history? How did she become—as many in her day called her—The Napoleon of the Women's Rights Movement?

I'm sure you've guessed the answer: She found her dharma and did it on purpose.

Susan B. Anthony began to sniff out her life's vocation in her late teens. From that point on, hers is a story of *the power of vocation itself to transform personality*—of dharma pulling toward its own realization. It is the story of a woman who understood her call and surrendered to it. Watch closely as I tell the story, and you will see Anthony's understanding of her own dharma come into focus—like a telescope at first only hazily focused on a distant star—and then in a series of consecutive corrections become sharper and clearer. Eventually the star—the dharma—comes in vividly, brilliantly, nuanced, alive.

—— 3 ——

In order to appreciate Susan B. Anthony's dharma story, we must first come to grips with the social and legal position of women in mid-nineteenth-century America. This is not going to be fun. The extent of women's disempowerment during that era—their almost total subjugation to men—is hard for us to wrap our heads around. Women living in America in the mid-1800s were the legal property of their husbands. A married woman had no right to property, no right to buy and sell real estate in her own name, no right to bequeath any property whatsoever to an heir. A married woman of the time had no right even to her own children. And, needless to say, she had no right to the vote.

As a result of her impoverished legal standing, a woman of that time lived in almost complete economic dependence upon her husband—or if she were "unfortunate" enough not to have a husband, upon her family. There were few roles for women outside the home. There was no social sphere in which women could come together to think and plan and dream on their own behalf. Indeed, outside the home women had very little independent existence whatsoever.

A telling story: Many women's gravestones at this time were etched with a revealing epitaph: "Here lies Mary Jones, *relict of the late Josiah Jones.*" Relict? A relict is, of course, the term used to refer to the surviving remnant of a natural phenomenon—or a surviving shard of an artifact. It is simply what is left over when the primary object is gone.

Women were in bondage of the most insidious sort—and there were no ready escape hatches from this social and political imprisonment. They had only two choices: marriage (which still amounted to legal serfdom), or spinsterhood (and the shame, loss of social esteem, and potential impoverishment that came with that "degrading station.")

Into such a world was Susan B. Anthony born.

Susan, however, was more fortunate than most. She was born a Quaker. As such, she found herself in a vastly different social milieu than other American girls—a world with at least a window open to other possibilities. Her family believed in absolute equality of the sexes. Her father was a staunch abolitionist, fighting for the emancipation of slaves in the decades just before the Civil War. And Susan was surrounded in her Quaker world by independent-thinking women. Independent-thinking women, and I hasten to say a certain *brand* of independent-thinking women—to wit: schoolteachers.

Schoolteachers were the role models for freedom-craving women of the day. There were very few roles in which a woman could claim social and economic independence, but teaching was one of them. Young Susan B. Anthony was impressed with the intelligence, education, and relative social autonomy of the teachers with whom she came into contact. From a young age, she knew only that she wanted to be like these women. And so, she became a teacher.

— 4 —

As young Susan B. Anthony educated herself about the world around her, she became aware of a paradox. She was living smack in the center of a culture shaped by Jacksonian democracy—a culture in which the *self-made man* was the national ideal. Everywhere there was talk of Emerson's spirit of self-reliance. People were reading Thoreau's new ideas about self-realization—many of them taken directly from the Bhagavad

Gita. "Man" was endowed with inalienable natural rights, it was believed, and it was his right to grow toward his unlimited potential. Anyone could grow up to be president!

Anyone, of course, except a woman. Susan became aware of the radical extent to which women were left out of this world of possibility. *Man was made for himself*—it was often said—*and woman for man!* "I was not made for man," Anthony would later declare flatly. "I was made for God. And I was made for myself."

By the time she reached young adulthood, Susan B. Anthony was aware that she had two choices: She could marry. Or she could be an old maid. Anthony would have neither. She was determined to reject the choice as society had defined it. Indeed she would stand the choices on their head. She would not marry, and she would make of the position of old maid something creative and new. Even in her midtwenties, Anthony had the spirit to declare: "These old Bachelors are nothing but a nuisance to a society but an Old Maid is the cleverest creature I ever saw."

By the age of twenty-five, Susan B. Anthony had made a conscious choice to remain single. "When I am crowned with all the rights, privileges, and immunities of a citizen," she declared, "I may give some consideration to this social institution [marriage]; but until then I must concentrate all of my energies on the enfranchisement of my own sex."

This was Susan B. Anthony's first dharma declaration. By her late twenties she had fully declared herself. *I must concentrate all of my energies on the enfranchisement of my own sex!* She had named and claimed her calling. Here is concentration of purpose. This declaration, as we shall see, unified her energy in extraordinary ways.

Naming her dharma allowed Susan to connect her life energy with an idea that was already very much in the atmosphere. It was the fantastic idea of the New True Woman. This idea was being written about in England, particularly in novels by Charlotte Brontë, and in poetry by Elizabeth Barrett Browning. Their riveting characters, Jane Eyre and Aurora Leigh, were New True Women of the type Susan had already imagined. Charlotte Brontë, dreaming of a powerful, but "plain and true" woman, had promised her sister Emily, "I will show you a heroine as plain and as small as myself, who shall be as interesting as any of yours." And voilà!: Jane Eyre!—the diminutive heroine who would be an inspiration to Anthony and millions of other men and women. Susan B. Anthony placed pictures of Charlotte Brontë and Elizabeth Barrett Browning over her bureau, and they would remain there for the rest of her life. At her request, these same pictures would hang on the wall above her coffin at her wake.

Susan wrote extensively about "the New True Woman." When she describes this "new being" her voice is electric with possibility: "The true woman will not be exponent of another, or allow another to be such for her. She will be her own individual self—do her own individual work—stand or fall by her own individual wisdom and strength . . . The old idea that man was made for himself and woman for him, that he is the oak, she the vine, he the head, she the heart, he the great conservator of wisdom principle, she of love, will be reverently laid aside with other long since exploded philosophies of the ignorant past."

Susan had a vision: Women will become acting subjects in their own destiny. This became her most fervently held personal and political manifesto. It was not just a vision for what might be in the future, but her blueprint for who she and her sisters in the struggle would be in the present. And it was in fact the very blueprint for who she would become.

— 5 —

By her late twenties, Susan B. Anthony had chosen her passion for social action over marriage as a vocation. She felt urgently called to *act*. She had begun her life of action by teaching, but the talented Anthony soon tired of teaching's routines. She wasn't bringing forth all that was within her, and she knew it. Teaching—as it was then practiced—was not a big enough palette for her capabilities. "I am tired of theory," she said. "I want to hear how we must *act* to have a happier and more glorious world."

Act she did. By her midtwenties, Susan had become deeply involved in temperance-reform activities. She saw clearly the direct connection between drunkenness and the abuse of women. The routine wife beatings she observed in her small community—most of them associated with male drunkenness—infuriated her. She spoke out. She became involved in the Women's Temperance Movement. And "Temperance" would be her first schooling in public action.

As soon as she began her life of action, Susan B. Anthony was presented with a challenge: how to marshal all of her life energy in support of her calling. One thing was perfectly clear: In order to fulfill her dharma, she would have to master the art of public speaking, she would have to learn how to unleash her power in full view of halls of angry men and skeptical women. This was a daunting challenge. It was almost unheard of for women to speak in public. It was considered an act of defiance and an unseemly betrayal of their proper role. Even Anthony's *right* to speak publicly was challenged by men at every turn. So for her to find her public-speaking voice she would have to summon every bit of determination and skill she could get her hands on. And she would have to overcome her considerable self-doubt.

Susan B. Anthony's path to her voice must have been thrilling to observe. She accomplished it through sheer guts and with many early failures. But several early successes pointed her in the right direction. One of her most dramatic early triumphs came in her relationship with the male-dominated temperance movement. In January 1852, Anthony attended a meeting called by the Sons of Temperance in Albany. She submitted her credentials along with the rest of the women, and took her place with them at the side of the hall, where it was understood that they (the women) were to remain silent—observing, and "learning from" the speeches of the men who dominated the organization.

Susan would have none of this. She rose to speak—in clear defiance of protocol. She was told by the male moderator that "the sisters were not invited here to speak but to listen and learn." She was enraged, and for the first time she allowed her fury to erupt publicly. She stormed out of the meeting, followed by a mob of sympathetic women. This was her first spontaneous protest action. Something inside had been liberated, and she would never be the same.

Emboldened by her first public act of defiance, Anthony organized a protest meeting, to which she pointedly invited only women—and also (one of her secret weapons throughout her life) the press. At the press conference, she announced that the protesting women would form their own independent organization. "We are heartily sick and tired of the round of demeaning encomiums which Gentlemen Temperance lecturers are pleased to lavish upon our sex," she exclaimed. And so, Susan B. Anthony's first organization, The Women's State Temperance Society, was born. Anthony did not stop there. She was on a roll: She immediately called a national Women's Temperance convention.

— 6 —

Susan B. Anthony decided that she would not be content to be a "good enough" public speaker. She must be great. Nothing else would fulfill her dharma. She became boldly single-minded in her practice. And she took on a coach: her closest friend, Elizabeth Cady Stanton—a masterful writer and speaker in various reform movements.

Stanton's coaching turned out to be phenomenal. She suggested that Susan "dress loose, take a great deal of exercise, and be particular about your diet and sleep sound enough, the body has a great effect on the mind." Cady might as well have been a yoga teacher, so much emphasis did she place on the body. Susan, still at times overcome by self-doubt, frequently tried to get Stanton herself to give the speeches she had written, but Stanton wisely refused: "I have no doubt a little practice will make you an admirable lecturer. I will go to work at once and write you the best lecture I can." And she did. Henceforth, the two would be a team—and a force to be reckoned with wherever they showed up.

A little practice will make you an admirable lecturer. Truer words were never spoken. Susan B. Anthony became a force of nature on the podium. She was Leontyne Price and Marian Anderson rolled into one. With her new skills giving her increasing self-confidence, she set about lecturing, organizing, petitioning, and raising money throughout New York. Suddenly, Susan B. Anthony was everywhere: She was speaking in churches, town halls, meeting rooms, individual homes. She was fast becoming that guided missile we spoke of earlier.

We have a number of written observations of Anthony's growth in her dharma. Clarina Howard Nichols, another women's rights advocate, wrote to Susan, "It is most invigorating to watch the development of a woman in the work for humanity: first, anxious for the cause and depressed with a sense of her own inability; next, partial success of timid efforts creating a hope; next, a faith; and then the fruition of complete self-devotion. Such will be your history." One could hardly have stated the progression more powerfully.

As Susan gathered and focused her energy, her strategy became clearer. Her biographer, Kathleen Barry, describes her unique method succinctly: "Take a concrete issue, such as intemperance; analyze the problem, formulate a specific demand . . . then urge women to take practical, confrontational and effective action that logically followed from her analysis of the issue. She was determined not only to act on behalf of women, but to mobilize women to act for themselves."

—— 7 ——

Susan's work gained in power. And it inevitably brought her face-to-face with the full extent of male domination. Many men who felt committed to the status quo found her presence—and her power—to be infuriating. The more successful she was, the more she had to face men's rage, and this routinely brought to her doorstep withering moments of public excoriation and every form of low personal attack.

Here is a typical newspaper rampage against Susan's work—and, really, her very existence. This article—one of hundreds of its ilk—specifically refers to Anthony's "agitation" for women's rights in marriage, and to a talk about the subject she gave one evening in Utica, New York. Keep in mind that the sentences come from a so-called "news story"—not an editorial—published the morning after her talk.

"With a degree of impiety which was both startling and disgusting, this shrewish *maiden* counseled the numerous wives and mothers present to separate from their husbands whenever they became intemperate, *and particularly not to allow the said husbands to add another child to the family* [probably no married advocate of woman's rights would have made this remark]. Think of such advice given in public by one who claims to be a *maiden lady*."

As part of her dharma training, Susan learned to toughen herself to these outbursts. She became famous for standing her ground with equanimity. There are dozens of fantastic stories of her facing down apoplectic men in public situations—usually winning the day with her calm, her

sense of humor, and her impressive composure under impossible circumstances. Angry men would simply come unglued in her presence.

Susan's diaries revealed the secret to her composure: She had early
on learned not to take any of these public excoriations personally. She
understood that they were *not about her in any personal sense*, but about
social and economic issues far larger than herself. As she said, "The mob
represents more than itself; it evidences that general masculine opinion
of woman, which condensed into law forges the chains which enslave
her."

Susan began to believe, as she often said, that in order to be effective,
"The important thing is to forget self." *Forget self.* Says Barry, "This was
the real philosophy behind her asceticism and the force that propelled
her through her campaigns. She cared little about her own comforts, nor
was she concerned with gaining personal rewards for her work. Success
was for the cause—for womankind—not for herself." For the rest of her
life, she would return again and again to this principle. "Forgetting self"
would become one of her principal mantras. She knew that "the work"
had energy and a power of its own, and was only undermined by any
hint of self-aggrandizement.

Everything she did—what she wore, how she lived—now came into
line with this principle. *Forget self.* She kept her physical needs very simple, which gave her more energy for her work. She dressed, as Stanton
had urged, simply and conservatively, so as not to draw attention to her
own person—always in dignified black. Susan loved colorful clothes.
But her dharma discipline required that she enjoy her few colorful
dresses at home and in her garden in Rochester. They were not for public work.

Barry describes it well: "Susan B. Anthony came to her platforms
with neither flourish nor flair. Always wearing a simple black dress with
a fitted 'basque waist' jacket, she walked with determined but not heavy
stride to the front of her audiences and stood very straight before them,
looked directly at them, and delivered her message. In Roundout, N. Y,
the papers reported that Anthony 'unattended and unheralded, quietly
glided in and ascended the platform.' She did not exhibit nervousness or
anxiety but instead was 'easy and self-possessed as a lady should always
be when performing a plain duty, even under 600 curious eyes.'"

The *Tao te Ching* says, "[The Master] doesn't glitter like a jewel . . . [but is] as rugged and common as a stone." This is a predictable characteristic of those who have matured into their dharma. We see it in every other character we've examined: Goodall, Thoreau, Whitman, and Frost. *Rugged and common as a stone.* As the inner life of the practitioner of dharma becomes more complex, the outer life becomes simpler.

Susan's audiences saw this. They felt it. They were moved by her simplicity, by the way in which her actions were in accord with her words. They were moved by the granite of her character, and her resolve. What her audiences felt was the power of someone living in the center of her dharma. We have evidence that even those who opposed her were moved. As one detractor admitted: "While we differ widely with Miss Anthony, both as regards the propriety of the calling she has assumed, and the notions of which she is advocate, we cheerfully accord to her credit, as a public speaker, much above mediocrity, expressing herself with clearness and many times with elegance and force."

Kathleen Barry captures it exactly: "She did not mince words but conveyed her message through the fiery passion of her convictions. If her audiences did not agree with her, she was too much the kind of character they respected to dismiss her even though she was a woman. The simplicity of her dress and the directness of her speech revealed a woman of common origins. She was a woman who had retained the simplicity of earlier life even as she had surpassed its limitations."

Susan B. Anthony *was* what she championed. She had become, through her own practice, the New True Woman.

— 8 —

For Susan B. Anthony, clarity about her vocation grew along with her actions in pursuit of dharma. That is to say, her actions themselves brought her increasing understanding of what was true. And they brought her, at midlife, to an epiphany: There could be no true success on the path to women's equality without the vote. Until women had the vote, they would always be the pawns of men in the political and social sphere. Any gains women made could quickly and easily be erased. And as Susan digested this truth, her calling became vividly clear. All of her energies must be devoted to the vote.

"Until women are made a balance of power—to be consulted, catered to, and bargained with, if you please—My one article of party creed—shall be that of woman suffrage—All other articles of party creeds shall be with me as a drop in the bucket—as compared with this vital one—hence I make it my whole party creed!!"

The telescope had now locked firmly onto the star. Now all of Anthony's actions came into alignment with her purpose. She refused to be distracted by other causes. She would, of course, remain passionately concerned about marriage laws, equal pay, coeducation. But she knew that the vote was the key to it all. Without the vote, none of the other gains could be sustained.

"Woman and her disfranchisement is all I know," she said.

Susan had matured into a visionary. She was supremely optimistic about the power of politics in American life. She knew that success was inevitable. She said, famously, "failure is impossible." But she knew, too, that it would take decades of work, consciousness-raising, education, and what she called "agitation" before the final goal would be achieved. And she knew that most likely the vote would not come in her lifetime. "Not in our day," she wrote, "but we must work on for future generations."

Susan B. Anthony understood a central teaching of the Bhagavad Gita: Complete devotion inexorably brings its own fulfillment. "When a person is devoted to something with complete faith," said Krishna to Arjuna, "I unify his faith in that form . . . Then, when his faith is completely unified, he gains the object of his devotion. In this way, every desire is fulfilled by me."

— 9 —

As she grew fully into her dharma, Susan saw that a great work can only be accomplished through a series of small acts. She called these small acts "subsoil plowing"—a wonderfully agricultural image from the daughter of a farmer. Later in life, Susan set about a campaign of education. She would lecture, raise consciousness among women, give them tools to speak, to organize. She would henceforward get women engaged through a kind of saturation-bombing approach. She moved tirelessly from town to town and city to city, preparing the ground for those whom she knew would come after her.

Once she found her dharma, it became the point of radiance around which all of her energies were organized. How she lived, ate, dressed, spoke, moved, thought, all began to move into orbit around *the work*. Her life itself took on the radiance and color of her central vision. This gave her life enormous power. But she understood that it was not *her* power. It was the power of the dharma.

Susan felt her own life's energy begin to connect with the bigger stream of social concern and suffering. "I believe our happiness is increased by yielding momentary self-gratification and doing all in our power to render others happy." In its most mature form, dharma inevitably puts the energies of self in the service of others—in the service of something bigger than self.

Susan's later life is exemplary of a central fact of dharma: It always involves the surrender of self to Self. In this surrender, action and awareness merge, time disappears, and the work is no longer "my" work, but "the work." The work becomes the path to God—the way of knowing the Divine essence.

Susan never denied the existence of God. But her beliefs were secularized and lodged in the world around her. When she was once asked, "Do you pray?" she responded, "I pray every single second of my life; not on my knees but with my work. My prayer is to lift women to equality with men. Work and worship are one with me."

—— 10 ——

Just three years before she died, Susan B. Anthony was attending—as she had for the previous forty years—the annual suffrage convention that was then being held in New Orleans. She was now eighty-three, and the honorary president of the organization. As she entered the hall, a thunderous ovation spontaneously erupted, and went on for many minutes.

Alarmed, Susan turned to her longtime lieutenant, Anna B. Shaw, and asked, "What has happened?"

Shaw replied, "You happened, Aunt Susan."

Anthony still looked puzzled.

"It's for you," explained Shaw to a dumbstruck Anthony. "The applause is for you."

"Nonsense," she shot back. "It's not for me. It's for the cause—The Cause."

— 11 —

"When a person is devoted to something with complete faith," said Krishna to Arjuna, "I unify his faith in that form."

Perhaps the most demanding practice in a life of dharma is the ongoing practice of unification—a process that Susan B. Anthony had mastered. Unification means simply that everything in your life must line up around the spine of your dharma. Eventually, everything that is *not* dharma must fall away—as it did in the life of Susan B. Anthony. Any life of dharma will demonstrate this principle.

Writing has been my own particular school for dharma, and it has taught me a lot about the challenges—and power—of the Bhagavad Gita's Doctrine of Unified Action. After all, when you look closely, you'll discover that writing a book is nothing more than a heroic act of unification. How does this work? Well, the book has a spine. A dharma. But you don't know what its dharma is until you begin to write it. Forget about all the things you said to yourself about your book at the beginning of the project—or what you told your editor, or what you wrote in your brilliant book proposal. No. The book has its own dharma, which will slowly reveal itself to you. And then you have a choice. You can choose the book's dharma. Or you can choose your *idea* of what the book should be. If you choose the latter, of course, the book will be a lousy book. It will have no power. If you choose the former—your book's authentic dharma—well, then you are really in deep trouble. Because you will have to bring absolutely everything you've got to the effort to manifest this book's true calling.

You'll hear the faint call of the book's dharma at first. And then you will have to practice listening very, very hard, day in and day out. You'll go down roads that you think are the dharma, and find them to be dead ends. You'll have to retrace your steps. You'll write wonderful chapters full of what you imagine to be wisdom and elegant sentences. And then you'll discover that they do not align with the book's dharma at all, and you will have to throw them on the floor of your writing room. You'll have to be relentless. Because the book will not fulfill its calling unless everything is lined up along the spine of the book's calling. Everything extra must go.

A life of dharma is exactly like a great yoga posture. Everything must be aligned around the spine. The dharma is a strict taskmaster. It will require you to *reach*—to work at your maximum potential. In order to do this, you will have to learn to take better care of yourself. You will have to sleep and eat properly. (In the case of a writer, you will have to stop abusing your mind with poorly written books.) You will probably have to create a regular schedule. And one day you'll realize you're in training like an Olympic athlete. But not any old training—a particular *kind* of training, the particular kind of training that will support *your* dharma and no one else's. The dharma itself will prescribe this training, and you will know it when you stumble onto it through trial and error. You'll know it by its results, because in moments when you're in proper training, you will feel yourself a channel for this book. You will have stepped aside somehow and let the book come through you. And this is an experience so far beyond any pleasure you've ever had that you will most definitely want more of it. And so you will henceforth be increasingly careful about your training regimen. You will give up that big bowl of ice cream before bed, because you know it'll leave you groggy in the morning. You want to be clear. For the book.

For brief moments during the writing, you will actually surrender to the book. In these moments of surrender, there is only the book. There is no you. There is no telling when these moments will arise. They may emerge on the worst morning of your writing career—after your girlfriend leaves you and the neighbor rear-ends your car. You know that if you don't go into training and suit up and show up every morning at your writing desk, these wonderful moments will in fact *never* happen. So you train as religiously as you can. Now you are hooked by dharma—by the magic of inaction in action.

You realize partway through (as Susan B. Anthony did in her life of dharma) that half measures will not work. You realize that a 70 percent investment of energy does not bring about a 70 percent book. It brings about a mediocre book. And then, really, what is the point? Does the world really need another half-assed book? So you see that you have to bring yourself 100 percent to the task.

Unification is the very soul of dharma. We see it in every life we've studied during this entire project. Thoreau streamlined his life in order to free his inner mystic. Frost became a farmer who farmed poetry. Goodall organized her life around her chimps. The degree of unification that you accomplish is the degree to which you're doing your dharma. "How we spend our days," says author Annie Dillard, "is, of course, how we spend our lives."

Once the mature Susan B. Anthony had fully organized her life around her dharma, she declared, as I have said, "Failure is impossible." She had grasped the central principle: As long as you are living your dharma fully—unified!—you cannot fail. Indeed, you have already succeeded.

SEVEN

Camille Corot:
Practice Deliberately

Bring into your mind's eye for a moment the most complicated sky you have ever seen. Perhaps you happened once over a ridge while hiking in the Vermont woods and came upon a strange show of orange and blue in the western sky. You and your buddy stopped in your tracks. Or maybe you came around a bend while driving out of the Pyrenees south into Spain, and you had to catch your breath upon the first sight of the endless pink mottled sky over the plain of Castile.

Now imagine that your deepest longing—your vocation—is to paint that sky. Imagine that you are so captivated by the play of nature and light that you must capture it in your net of paints and brushes—render its mystery palpable on the plain white canvas. It is no small task. How will you do it?

Such was the experience—and the dilemma—of Jean-Baptiste-Camille Corot, a French painter of the mid-nineteenth century who became, over the course of a long career, one of the greatest landscape painters of all time.

Some of us perhaps flirted briefly with Camille Corot in that one required course on the history of Western art that we took in school. We then forgot him. It's easy to do. Corot did not live a dramatic life. There were no sexual scandals or flamboyant mistresses. There were no screaming fights or flaming rivalries with other artists. Only the long life of a dedicated craftsman.

Corot did not seek fame. In fact, he was remarkably immune to it. He once said that he hoped his paintings would be celebrated but that he would be forgotten. Corot lived for his work. He was a kind of artist-monk. He never married. In fact, he declared early that his life would be dedicated to art, and there would be little room for wives or mistresses.

Corot was an artist's artist. Other painters of the time adored him, watched him closely, learned from him. They also copied him brazenly—and sometimes they privately hated him. In 1897, when Claude Monet was nearly sixty, he was viewing a retrospective of Impressionist paintings, including canvases by Corot. The well-known art critic Raymond Koechlin was at Monet's side, and declared aloud how wonderful it was to have "so many great works of art gathered together." Monet replied, "There is only one master here—Corot. Compared to him, the rest of us are nothing." Then he added, "This is the saddest day of my life."

When I accidentally stumbled into an exposition of Corot's work at the National Gallery in Washington, D.C., in 1996, I had entirely forgotten who the man was. I had found my way into an exposition called *In the Light of Italy: Corot and Early Open-Air Painting*. It traced the development of the European school of open-air landscape painting of which Corot was a granddaddy. There were quite a few canvases by The Master. They took my breath away.

How had I missed the genius of this giant of Western art? Why hadn't pictures of his fantastic work drawn me to him before? Well, these were the kinds of paintings whose power could only be hinted at in photographs. In India it is claimed that certain adept yogis cannot be photographed. The power of their body's energy is too subtle. So, too, apparently, Corot's canvases. Seen live, they pulsed with a subtle inner light.

These paintings were not "about" anything. They were not "representations" of nature. They were not copies of nature. They were, as Thoreau would have said, "the thing itself." (Emerson exhorted Thoreau to let his work so live and breathe that every sentence would be its own evidence!) Frost said of his poems: "They are an idea of an idea of an idea." Corot's paintings, likewise, were an idea of an idea of an idea: Condensed. Coiled. Alive.

—— 2 ——

Jean-Baptiste-Camille Corot was born in Paris in 1796 into a family of genteel merchants. His mother ran one of the most elegant dressmaking salons in the Rue du Bac—a fashionable district of the French capital. His father ran the business side of the salon, and hoped—not unreasonably, one imagines—that his only son, Camille, would eventually join him in the family venture.

This was not to be. Young Corot had no interest in business. He loved to draw and paint, and was best known at the salon for ruining expensive pieces of fabric with his paint-stained hands and dirty drawing supplies.

As a schoolboy, Corot had had a fortuitous encounter with a landscape painting that changed his life. He described the painting, which he had seen in the Louvre Museum: ". . . the artist had captured for the first time the effects that had always touched me when I discovered them in nature and that were rarely painted. I was astonished. His small picture was for me a revelation. I discerned its sincerity and from that day I was firm in my resolution to become a painter."

Corot saw in this painting his own future. After his first encounter, the boy simply haunted the Louvre. He stood open-mouthed at the paintings of Claude Lorrain, one of France's greatest landscape painters. Eventually, the attendants at the Louvre galleries would have to physically move him on.

Corot is often described as "a dreamy youth"—with an enchantingly good nature. He spent much of his time hanging around his mother's dressmaking studio, playing the violin, and singing for the sewing girls while they worked. Corot's father thought he was just plain lazy. By the time he had reached twenty-six, his father had given up hope in the boy's future. He was, in his father's eyes—and in the eyes of his sterner teachers—a failure. One thinks, when hearing these descriptions, of young Henry David Thoreau, or of Walt Whitman at practically any age. What do we make of this list of losers and ne'er-do-wells who become great exemplars of dharma?

Corot's father—at wit's end—finally agreed to let him paint ("to pursue your crazy adventure") on the condition that he come back to the family business when he (inevitably) discovered that painting was no kind of a life.

Corot was so delighted with his father's decision to let him paint that he burst into tears and embraced his austere parent with both arms. Straightaway he set up an easel on the towpath next to the Seine, and began to paint. He would continue to paint until his dying day, at seventy-seven. (His father never really did catch on: When Corot, at midlife, was presented by the French government with the prestigious Légion d'Honneur for his landscapes, his father asked a friend, "Do you really think he has talent?")

As it turned out, Corot was not the dreamy youth he appeared to be. He was dead serious. He began to study painting intensively—initially with his good friend Achille Etna Michallon, already a well-respected teacher. Young Corot also did the usual practice of copying the masters—in the studio, and in the Louvre. But from the beginning he was enchanted by painting *outdoors,* especially in the forests of Fontainebleau, the seaports along Normandy, and the villages west of Paris such as Ville d'Avray, where his parents kept a charming country house.

Naturally, Corot studied the masters—especially his early heroes, Claude Lorrain and John Constable. But he spent as much time as he could sketching and painting in nature. In the final analysis, "nature," he said, "was my best teacher." He would later instruct his own students to forget all they had been taught in the gallery, and let nature teach them. *Observe carefully! Paint what you see! Paint what you feel!* "Do not follow others," Corot exhorted. "He who follows is always behind. You must interpret Nature with entire simplicity and according to your personal sentiment, altogether detaching yourself from what you know of the old masters or of contemporaries. Only in this way will you do work of real feeling."

—— 3 ——

Every couple of weeks I climb the three flights of creaky old wooden stairs to the office of Lonny Jarrett, my acupuncturist in nearby Stockbridge, Massachusetts. The rich smell of 150-year-old wood in Lonny's office building always reminds me of the smell of my family's summer house—built in 1893 by my great-grandfather, and not changed substantially since. The floors in Lonny's third-floor garret are so slanted that the bathroom door closes itself. There is something honest and welcoming about this space: "rough-hewn as a stone."

In Lonny's office, one entire wall of bookshelves is stacked with yellowing esoteric books written in ancient Chinese dialects. His shelves are replete with exotic-looking medicine jars, formulas, and herbs, some bound in cloth and stamped with wax seals. There are wall charts with images of human bodies crisscrossed with red lines of *qi,* or energy. This is the enchanting world of Lonny Jarrett—a handsome, dark-haired, intelligent-looking man in his late fifties.

Lonny greets me, and we go through our little ritual. I sit down in the comfortable chair in his treatment room and hold up one arm. He holds my wrist gently while his fingers move oh-so-subtly around the area of my artery—while I stare contentedly off into the middle distance. Lonny is checking my pulses. I find this all very pleasurable. His touch is warm, soothing, reassuring. But what does he detect with his fingers? What secrets is my body giving up to him? And how does he know how to read them? He asks to see my tongue. (Later, in the car, I look at my own tongue in the rearview mirror. What does it mean, I wonder?)

Sometimes I think Lonny is just making this all up. Perhaps nothing is *really* happening in these mysterious exams. They're a scam. A little ritual meant to inspire confidence in me. (There is a sucker born every minute.) I wonder: Is *everything* that happens in Lonny's exotic world really just placebo? Is there an active ingredient other than his caring?

What precisely *does* Lonny feel when he checks my pulse? Clearly (unless it *is* mumbo jumbo) he is recognizing patterns of which I am entirely unaware. He speaks a language I do not understand. (When I attended my first faculty dinner party in college, I remember several of the older professors talking about wine as if each wine were an entirely new country—an exotic place with its own hills and valleys, smells, character. Huh? Was this wine-connoisseur stuff really just complete fantasy? Why couldn't I taste that "hint of oak" that seemed so perfectly obvious to everyone else?)

After Lonny takes my pulse, I know what comes next. I take off my shirt and roll up my pant legs, take off my socks, and get up on the treatment table. Now Lonny inserts the needles. Is he making this up, too? Does it really matter where they go? Do the "points" he "treats" really correspond to those lines on the poster displayed on the wall? He inserts the needles into points with exotic names: Reaching Heaven, Spirit's Door, Jade Pillow.

It is during this part of the experience that I know for sure that this is not mere voodoo. Because when the needles are inserted, I feel the energy grid depicted on those wall hangings light up in my own body. With certain treatments, I go into a delightful altered state. This state sometimes lasts for hours (and in rare cases, days). At times, an acupuncture treatment with Lonny is like the very best drug experience you've ever had (or read about)—and it is all perfectly legal.

But I discovered over time that there was something much more profound going on here than just altered states. Indeed, over the course of months, I began to perceive some inner shift that I can only describe as leading me to a new state of wholeness—mental clarity, physical vitality, enhanced awareness. What was this magic?

—— 4 ——

Camille Corot, the landscape painter, and Lonny, the acupuncturist, are separated by two hundred years and an ocean of cultural differences. And yet, they inhabit the same sphere: the sphere of mastery. One knows when one is in its presence. One can simply *feel* it. The master may be utterly like the rest of us in every other way, but *in his own domain he sees more deeply.* He perceives aspects of reality that are entirely outside our perceptual range. Thoreau, through his mastery of the forest, began to perceive aspects of the flora and fauna around Concord that no one had ever recorded. Jane Goodall, over the course of decades, learned to perceive the subtle language of the chimpanzee. Robert Frost tuned in to the ineffable syntax, rhythm, and song of the spoken word of New England—and mapped it in a way no one ever had.

Mastery. What is it, precisely? And what is its relationship to dharma?

Within the past decade, serious research into the characteristics of mastery has unearthed a surprising fact: Mastery is almost never the result of mere talent. It is, rather, the blending of The Gift with a certain quality of sustained and intensive effort—a quality of effort that has now come to be called "deliberate practice."

Jean-Baptiste-Camille Corot and Lonny Jarrett have dharma stories that perfectly exemplify deliberate practice, and the potent mix of *giftedness* and *effort*—fire and gasoline—that, over extended periods of time, may burst forth into a bonfire of mastery.

— 5 —

When Camille Corot was twenty-nine years old—and well on his way to becoming a professional painter—he left France for a painting trip to Italy. A brief apprenticeship in Italy was part of the grand tour for all aspiring artists in those days. But Corot's experience went well beyond the norm. He would stay in Italy for three years—moving back and forth between Rome and Naples, between the woods at Papigno and the banks of the Nera River—and would produce hundreds of sketches, drawings, and fully completed canvases. His paintings from this period would later be recognized as great early masterpieces. His efforts in Italy would be the crucible in which young Corot would begin his journey toward mastery and create the discipline that would take him to the pinnacle of landscape painting. What happened to him in Italy that transformed him into a master? And what set him apart from his many painter friends there who did not achieve mastery?

It all began with a quandary. From the very beginning, Italy provided young Corot with what he feared would be an insurmountable challenge: the Italian light. This damned Italian light was subtly but infuriatingly different from the light in France—and painting it required Corot to dig deep into his slim skill set (and his considerable resolve). Early on in his Italian adventure he wrote home to his friends:

"You could not imagine the weather we have at Rome. Here it is now a month that I am awakened each morning by a blaze of sunlight that strikes the wall of my room. In short, the weather is always beautiful. On the other hand, I find this brilliant sunlight dispiriting. I feel the complete impotence of my palette. Console your poor friend, who is thoroughly tormented to see his efforts in painting so miserable, so sad, beside the dazzling scene before his eyes. There are days, truly, when I would throw the whole lot to the devil."

Corot set to work to master this challenge. What followed were three years of intensive growth in his practice of capturing the subtle effects of light on stone and field—and an altogether different play of sky and shadow than he had known. He had an early breakthrough: After some initial investigation, Corot realized that the intense Mediterranean light did not actually strengthen bright colors as he had thought. Rather, it *bleached* them. He discovered, through systematic experimentation, that he could add white lead to his pigments, and thereby achieve a more accurate representation of the sun-drenched landscapes. But this was just the beginning. Breakthrough followed breakthrough as he bore down on his challenge.

In his attempts at mastery, Corot did something that was strictly forbidden by several of his teachers. He returned to the same scene day after day—and at several different times of day—attempting both to *see* and to *paint* the subtle variations of these scenes as they changed with the weather and the light. The most famous of these studies is a trio of finished paintings called *View in the Farnese Gardens*. For three weeks in March of 1826, Corot painted all day—every day—from the Palatine Hill in Rome. In the morning, he faced east-southeast toward the church of San Sebastiano in Palatino; at midday he faced east-northeast, toward the Colosseum; and in the afternoon he looked north toward the Forum.

In this series of paintings from the Palatine Hill, one can see something altogether new emerge in Corot's work. He was learning, through practice, to capture astonishing subtleties of light and shadow—and a sense of the soul of the hour. These paintings are alive. There is both movement and quiet, and a kind of inner pulsation of energy. They are the fruit of a new quality of attention that the artist was developing. Corot was systematically training his attention to see more deeply into his subjects—to see them, and to master them.

With this series, Corot began to attract attention among the scruffy lot of landscape painters with whom he socialized every evening at Caffè Greco in Rome. Caruelle d'Aligny, one of the great young painters who was carefully observing Corot's progress in Rome, announced to the assembled landscapists at their mutual hangout one evening: "Corot is our master."

Why did Corot stand out from the crowd of his painter friends? Was it inborn talent? Genius? No. It was the *quality of his practice.* He was engaging in what some contemporary students of optimal performance now call "deliberate practice." Deliberate practice is not just a laborious repetition of the tasks of artistry. It is, rather, a kind of sustained engagement in the work that is *aimed specifically at understanding and improving the work.* It is an intentional breaking down of the tasks of any domain into smaller and smaller components to see precisely how they work. And it results in steady and incremental improvements in performance.

Corot was engaging in deliberate practice of his art. On the Palatine Hill he had intentionally given himself an assignment to improve his capacity to capture difficult and subtle changes in light. He looked systematically at how he was mixing colors. At how he was composing scenes. At where he was standing. At how he was applying the paint. He made careful observations of his work as he went, and then examined it again every night with his friends, using their eyes to help him evaluate things he may have missed. He was working intentionally for new and more accurate, or more interesting, effects.

Corot's finished work from this early Italian period has a lightness and ease that is disarming. But in spite of its apparent offhandedness it was actually very carefully composed. Corot developed a habit of working precisely. He stayed longer at each scene than the other artists. He persevered in his work from each station. He wrote in one of his notebooks: "One must be severe in the face of nature and not content oneself with a hasty sketch. How many times in reviewing my drawings have I regretted not having had the courage to stay at it half an hour more! . . . One must not allow indecision in a single thing."

Says critic Peter Galassi: "Many of Corot's best open-air paintings . . . possess a freshness and buoyancy that is closer to athletic grace than to intellectual deliberation. The study is a document of the liveliness—one is tempted to say, the abandon—of its own making. But like the athlete,

Corot did not depend on natural talent alone. A deep effort of preparation and concentration lay behind his spirited performance."

Here was the key to Corot's development: the discovery of the compelling fruit of "deliberate practice."

— 6 —

Several years ago, Lonny Jarrett and I had lunch together at a café near his office. I asked Lonny how he got into acupuncture. In a leisurely fashion, Lonny laid out for me a riveting dharma story—a story that exemplifies many of the same principles we find in Corot.

Even as a child, Lonny had a gift. He was curious about the mind. He wanted to understand consciousness. ("Consciousness?" I thought. Did I even know the word when I was a kid?) Eventually, as part of his quest to understand the mind, Lonny had enrolled in graduate school in neurobiology—assuming that an examination of the brain would bring him closer to a grasp of the elusive facts of consciousness. He got himself far enough up to his elbows in neurobiology to discover that this science was not, alas, really about consciousness at all. He gradually began to see that consciousness itself was not actually located in the brain.

Lonny began to throw his net wider. At one point in his search, he took a ten-week course in Chinese medicine and diagnosis. In this course the teacher gave a brief overview of pulse taking, and began to teach about the energy fields of the body (those wall charts I see in Lonny's office). One episode from this ten-week course stood out vividly, and Lonny brightened as he told it.

During the last week of the course, he and his classmates and their teacher sat around in a circle. Each student would stand up and talk for a minute or two. Then everyone else in the circle would diagnose that particular student—making an effort to describe his precise energy type and his probable physical strengths and vulnerabilities seen from an Eastern, whole-systems perspective. To his surprise, Lonny nailed every diagnosis—stunning the teacher and the rest of the students as well. He discovered that he could rely on an intuitive part of his mind—a gift he hadn't even known he had. He found to his delight that this form of medicine used all of him—all of his gifts. And he came to believe that Chinese medicine had everything that was missing from Western medicine.

"Sitting around that circle," said Lonny, "something shifted in me." He realized that while neurobiology sees consciousness as a by-product of neural functioning, Chinese medicine considers the entire material universe to be an outward manifestation of consciousness. He had finally found the domain in which he could explore consciousness itself. He soon signed up for a course in acupuncture, and eventually took the entire program. The rest is history. Lonny has gone on to write several important books in the field, and to become a master practitioner.

While he was doing his coursework, Lonny met Leon Hammer—a distinguished scholar and practitioner of Chinese medicine. Hammer, a psychologist, was teaching the first real psychological presentation of Chinese medicine in the United States. When Lonny graduated from the course, he discovered that Hammer lived just an hour north of him. He invited Hammer to be his mentor, and proceeded to work intensively with him for the next decade.

During this ten-year apprenticeship, Leon and Lonny saw hundreds of patients together. Sometimes they would spend two hours taking just one patient's pulses. Then they spent another two hours discussing in detail what they discovered in those pulses—precisely *how* they discovered it, and what it meant. Altogether, these two men would spend an astonishing four hours on each patient. In the early phase, Lonny says, it required a tremendous amount of concentration for him to perceive the subtleties of the various pulses. In the process, he could feel himself learning, stretching, improving. It was intense. It was difficult. But it was at times exhilarating. There were plateaus when nothing seemed to be happening. And then there were moments of breakthrough.

I was fascinated to hear Lonny describe how, often, just when he thought he had reached a solid ground of understanding, some new insight would pull the ground out from under him—and he'd feel disoriented, as if everything he thought he knew was dropping away. In these times, Lonny would doubt himself: Am I hypnotizing myself into believing a complex metaphysic that is actually *baseless*? he wondered. (This, of course, exactly paralleled my own early experience of doubt about acupuncture.) Then, inevitably, a bigger picture would emerge—more complete than before—and Lonny would gain higher ground in his practice.

Lonny described the way in which mastery begins to show itself. "You begin to study, and for a while you just don't get it. You don't think you know anything. And then one day, you get a whiff of something. There it is! You perceive a pulse. Then you begin to feel for it everywhere. On your wife, your kids, your friends. Then, after a while, your teacher points you to a deeper pulse, and at first you don't get *that*. You're frustrated. But you hang in there. Eventually you begin to get a glimmer of this new pulse, this more subtle pulse. And suddenly, you're on a new plateau. And that's how it goes." Just so. This is deliberate practice.

— 7 —

The scientific investigation of deliberate practice began with the unique contribution of researchers K. Anders Ericsson and Neil Charness, whose article "Expert Performance: Its Structure and Acquisition" is a standard text of the field. As it turns out, "expert practice" (or performance that leads to what Ericsson calls "eminent performance") requires certain factors, all of which Corot and Lonny had stumbled onto—either through the course of formal instruction, or as a result of their own deep motivation to learn. These are the factors required for expert practice, paraphrased here from Ericsson's work:

- Sustained and intensive practice of a skill for several hours a day
- Practice with the specific intention of *improving*, not just repeating
- Practice that is sustained in this manner for a matter of years—in most cases as many as ten years
- Practice that includes a particular mechanism by which the results of practice can be *evaluated* and *improved upon* in future sessions
- The intentional development of sophisticated feedback loops—teachers and colleagues commenting on progress; other pairs of expert eyes on the work

- Appropriate care paid to the essential ingredient of "recovery time" so that there is energy to engage in the same intense practice again the next day
- A considerable amount of time spent within the so-called "domain of the task." For Corot, for example, this meant hanging out with other painters—talking about his art, talking about trends in art, getting support for the lifestyle of the artist.

For Corot, for Lonny, and for all masters, deliberate practice is really about the *training of attention.* It involves learning to sustain attention on a complex task, and to come back to that task over and over again; to stay with it just a little bit longer each time. (Remember Corot's telling comment: "How often I had wished I had stayed longer!")

Most of young Corot's contemporaries in Italy had not yet stumbled onto these secrets. They drew or painted views just once. They were under the common misapprehension that it is the sheer *volume* of practice that creates mastery. Corot, however, saw that it was not the volume, but the *quality* of his practice. He had to try to make every canvas better than the last—and he worked to understand *why* it was better.

Remember our friend Hokusai? *Every dot and stroke will be alive!* Hokusai did precisely this kind of practice in his masterful *Thirty Views of Mt. Fuji,* of which the aforementioned *Great Wave* is a part. Claude Monet was doing this, too, when he painted eighteen canvases of the façade of the Rouen Cathedral, minutely recording all its variations in color from dawn to sunset.

— 8 —

Deliberate practice is really a kind of sophisticated *attentional training.* It bears fruit when *attention begins to penetrate the object of its interest in an entirely new way.* With sustained practice, the master's perception of the object becomes refined. Aspects of the object that had previously been out of perceptual range begin to come into perceptual range. Eventually, for example, Corot began to observe subtle aspects of color and light in the Italian countryside that others simply did not see. The quality of his *perception* was refined in parallel with his skill at capturing it.

This refinement of attention is a central component of mastery. Technically, it is called "the development of pattern recognition." With practice, the master begins to see patterns that others cannot yet see. Lonny begins to see energy patterns in the pulse. Thoreau begins to see plants in the Concord woods that no one had previously noticed or cataloged. (The last great unfinished work of Thoreau's life was a mammoth classification system of nature; he was seeing entirely new patterns of flora, of seasonal change, of fauna.) Beethoven—as we shall see in a forthcoming chapter—in his late work began to see patterns and opportunities in the sonata form that no one had seen before.

Experts gradually learn to see their object of study with something more than ordinary vision. They see the object, as it were, "fresh." In contemplative practice, this is sometimes called "beginner's mind." This fresh seeing involves two related components: First, a master sees the *parts* of the object in enormous detail—in much more detail than normal. But at the same time—and most important—he sees these parts in their relationship to *the whole. He sees both the parts and the whole at the same time.* When a chess master looks at a board during a game, he sees hundreds of potential individual moves (many more than the average player sees) but more important, he sees them in relationship to the outcome of the overall game. This gives the individual moves heightened *meaning.*

It is well known that expert meditators develop the capacity to see life in slow motion, observing objects (including their own thoughts) in minute detail, as if seeing every individual frame of a movie. It turns out that masters in every field develop the same capacity. Master baseball players, for example, when at bat, see the ball coming at them as if in slow motion—even though the ball is actually traveling 90 miles an hour. Not only can the master batter see the ball in "individual frame" detail, but he can at the same time see the *meaning of those details.* How low is the ball to the ground? Over what quadrant of the plate will it pass? Is it spinning? In what direction? How will all of this detail influence my decision about how and where I want to hit the ball? This is mastery.

The great Japanese-American conductor Seiji Ozawa almost always conducts great symphonies without a score. He knows each individual moment in the score in great detail, of course. But he also *sees that individual moment in the context of the whole symphony.* So, in each moment, he holds both the part and the whole in his mind.

Corot developed precisely this kind of mastery. His students observed that as he matured, he appeared to visualize the completed painting as he approached a fresh canvas. He was famous for running his hand lightly over a fresh canvas, feeling it, making love to it, as it were. He would imagine an ideal structure in his mind's eye, placing objects in just the right relationship to one another. Indeed, by all accounts, he would not start a canvas until he had seen it whole.

Lonny has a remarkably similar story to tell about his practice of acupuncture and Chinese medicine. After I had known him for a while, he confided to me that he "knows exactly how to treat a person as soon as the person comes into the room." There are so many cues visible to his naked and knowing eye, that he does not really need to take pulses. He takes pulses only to confirm the hunches that are already forming in his mind, and because it builds patients' confidence that he is not actually just performing voodoo. This confidence emerges from the degree of detail Lonny is able to perceive about a patient by merely touching his wrist for a moment or two. Lonny's perception has now become so refined that he sees those energy grids, depicted in his wall hangings, come alive in each patient who walks into his treatment room.

The capacity to know a certain domain of the world in such depth appears to us ordinary mortals as a kind of supernormal power. It seems like magic. It is not magic at all, of course, but simply the inevitable result of sustained concentration on an object of intense interest.

Any one of us can discover these principles—and these capacities—in our own domain, whether it be stamp collecting or gardening or selling insurance. I have stumbled onto most of these principles in my own domain—writing. As it turns out, Ericsson and his friends have studied writers, and have a great deal to say about the subject. Great writers, they discovered (not surprisingly) see a manuscript whole—just as a chess master sees a chessboard whole. Even when working on details, the master writer always holds in mind the entire scope of her argument. She sees the parts in relationship to the whole. Ericsson found that while revising manuscripts, for example, expert writers focus on global problems, while novice writers focus on local problems. Novice writers spend the bulk of their time assessing whether they are using the correct word or phrase, or in evaluating the structure of a sentence. They become easily lost in the details, and lose the global view of the whole argument. In contrast, expert writers constantly evaluate the form or shape of their argument. Expert writers focus on making sure that their global meaning is communicated through the words and sentences. The meaning is primary, and every word, sentence, and paragraph in a polished work must support this meaning.

Both Lonny's and Corot's stories help us make sense of mastery as heightened pattern recognition. The process of pattern recognition continues to deepen throughout the career of a master, until the more obvious surface patterns dissolve to reveal even more subtle patterns underneath. Later in his life, Thoreau saw so deeply into summer's shades and movements that he began to perceive the beginnings of autumn in the middle of the summer. He could tell you the precise day in midsummer when autumn began.

An understanding of this process is important because it helps us appreciate the profound pleasure of mastery, and why it leads to a sense of fulfillment in life. The pleasures of mastery are not what we usually assume them to be. They do not center around the *control* of one's particular domain—an inference one might understandably take from the word "master" itself. They center, rather, around *knowing*. It is the profound pleasure in knowing the world more deeply that creates authentic fulfillment. This is what dharma is all about. Neither Lonny nor Corot is motivated by control—or by other extrinsic factors like money and fame. There is a much, much deeper pleasure: the pleasure in knowing the world.

—— 9 ——

Corot returned from Italy a changed man. He had seen the light—both literally and figuratively—and this *seeing* gave rise to the famous dharma declaration he made from Italy in August 1826. He wrote home to his parents: "All I really want to do in life, and without deviation, is to paint landscapes." Here was the declaration of an artist who had had an early taste of the pleasures of *knowing his object*. He would spend the rest of his life pursuing this experience.

When Corot returned to France after his Italian tour, he began to develop the schedule that he would follow for the rest of his life. Every morning he climbed the four flights of stairs to his studio on the rue Paradis-Poissonnière. (Throughout his over fifty years of working life, he boasted that he reached his studio every morning at three minutes before eight.)

Corot's vision continued to deepen throughout his mature years, and he painted constantly until the end of his life. He was a famously happy man. And he describes the key to his happiness thus: "Ceaseless work, either executing or observing," he wrote in one of his sketchbooks. And he added: "An invulnerable conscience." Corot was a fulfilled man if ever there was one.

Mastery gave Corot everything he wanted in life. He was filled up with beauty—and with a deep knowledge of nature. And out of this fulfillment, he became a wonderfully generous man—indeed, a person of positively fabled generosity. Throughout his life, Corot was personally frugal. He famously said, "I could be gay on a loaf of bread." But he loved to give to others. Indeed, as he grew older, his greatest pleasure was to give. Late in life, when he became a wealthy man as a result of the success of his art, he gave away much of his fortune. In 1871, he gave 10,000 francs to the poor of Paris. He bought a cottage for fellow painter Honoré Daumier, who had not been as successful as he. He also regularly supported the widow of his great friend, the painter Jean-François Millet.

Great masters of any domain (even our stamp collector) inevitably discover the truth that *to know the world is the chiefest delight in life*. I do not mean to know it *cognitively*. I do not mean to "have knowledge about it." It is not that kind of knowledge that frees. Rather, it is direct knowledge of the world—*penetrating underneath the appearance of things to their essence, to their soul*. For when one penetrates to the soul of any object, one also penetrates one's own soul. This is a central principle of the Bhagavad Gita, and one that Krishna teaches over and over again:

The whole world is inside each person, each being, each object. To know any *part* of the world deeply, intimately, is to know the whole.

Each of us, then, must find our own particular domain—that little corner of the world in which we can drill for gold. For the acupuncturist it is knowing the body through the language of Chinese medicine. For the painter, it is knowing the world through paint and the canvas. For the writer, it is knowing the world through words. ("When you write, you lay out a line of words," says Pulitzer Prize-winning American author Annie Dillard. "The line of words is a miner's pick, a wood-carver's gouge, a surgeon's probe. You wield it, and it digs a path you follow. Soon you find yourself deep in new territory.")

We each pick our own path. Thoreau does it through knowing nature. Goodall, through the contemplation of chimps. Whitman saw it in the faces of his soldiers. Susan B. Anthony said her work was her worship—her way of knowing. Her way of getting close to the beating heart of the world. A taste of this knowledge—the knowledge of the sacred, the numinous—pulls us on— and this taste contains within it more satisfaction than all the honors the world has to give.

—— 10 ——

Finally, as Krishna teaches Arjuna, when you come to know the world, you also come to love it. It's simple: You love what you know deeply. This was obviously true for Corot. The act of painting became an act of joy for him throughout his long life. He never tired of it. For Corot, painting was a part of his love affair with nature. When he was seventy-one years old he wrote: "All must be governed by your love of nature. By what you feel, by what you experience in nature. When in July, I bury my nose in a hazelbush, I shall be fifteen years old."

Eventually Camille Corot painted not just nature, but his *love of nature*. This is what I had experienced at the exposition at the National Gallery. The paintings are not *representations* of nature, but are nature itself—are, as Emerson suggested, not a reference to something else but are "things in themselves"—with living souls. This is why they cannot be accurately reproduced in a photograph.

At the age of seventy-seven, before he died, Corot said, "You have no idea of the things I could paint now. I see what I have never seen before. New tints, new skies, new horizons." He concluded: "I go on hoping that there will be painting in heaven."

After his death, 5,000 art students wore black crêpe on their arms for a year "in memory of Papa Corot."

Camille Corot, in following his dharma, had truly brought the "heaven" of painting down to earth.

PART IV

The Third Pillar:
"Let Go of the Fruits"

Krishna and Arjuna are now deep into their conversation about dharma. Krishna, as we have seen, has begun the "sacred dialogue" with two primary teachings: First—look to your dharma. Then—do it full out! Now he presents Arjuna with a third and most puzzling lesson: "Let go of the fruits of your actions."

To which Arjuna replies, essentially, "Huh?"

"You have the right to work," says Krishna to his bewildered student, "but never to the fruit of work."

Arjuna will struggle with this teaching more than with any other. Indeed, this lesson is so slippery that Krishna will have to reiterate it over and over again to Arjuna throughout the dialogue: "You should never engage in action for the sake of reward, nor should you long for inaction. Perform work in this world, Arjuna, as a man established within himself—without selfish attachments, and alike in success and defeat."

In this third lesson, Krishna is transmitting to Arjuna one of the most brilliant discoveries of the ancient yoga tradition: the power of nonattachment. Give yourself entirely to your work, yes. *But let go of the outcome. Be alike in success and defeat.* Krishna is emphatic on this point: You cannot devote yourself fully and passionately to your dharma *without* engaging this principle.

Why? Over the course of hundreds of years of practice, yogis had discovered that *clinging to outcome has a pernicious effect on performance.* Clinging (or grasping) of any kind disturbs the mind. And this disturbed mind, then, is not really fully present to the task at hand. It is forever leaning forward into the next moment—grabbing. And, not being present for the moment, it cannot fully devote its powers to the job at hand.

We find ourselves, at this point, right back to our old friend, doubt. Grasping, it turns out, is just another form of doubt. Grasping, or craving, or clinging to a particular outcome *splits the mind from the present moment.* The mind that is constantly evaluating—"How am I doing?" or "How am I measuring up?" or "Am I winning or losing?"—is the divided mind.

Krishna speaks about this with vivid psychological insight: "Those who are motivated only by desire for the fruits of action," he teaches, "are miserable, for they are constantly anxious about the results of what they do." The yoga tradition systematically investigated this anxiety about outcome. It found that grasping has three pernicious effects on the mind. They are: first, disturbance; then, obscuration; and finally, separation.

This analysis is really one of the most useful discoveries of the yoga tradition. Let's look at it more closely.

First, grasping "disturbs" the mind. Anyone can see this simply by observing the mind and body when caught up in a state of craving. Try this: Sit down to meditate when you're caught up in a moment of craving for food or sex. Notice the quality of the mind. Crazy! One can see that the mind is stirred up, restless—or, as yogis would say, "overheated."

Second, grasping in any form is said to "obscure" the mind. What does this mean? Simply that when the mind is caught up in grasping it *does not see clearly.* It is obscured. This, too, is easy to observe in everyday life. When the mind is craving a particular object or outcome, that object looks "all good" to the mind. When the mind is craving, say, a bowl of chocolate fudge brownie ice cream, the ice cream seems all good. In that moment of grasping, we do not see that there are perhaps pros and cons to this bowl of ice cream. (Perhaps we're committed to a diet, or we're not eating sugar, or we are kept awake by chocolate, or we are in serious trouble with our cholesterol.) In a moment of grasping, the mind does not see the gray areas. No! It adopts a kind of tunnel vision toward the object. Ice cream! All good! I want it! The mind caught up in craving does not make discerning choices. In these moments we are said to be *obscured*.

And third, the mind caught up in a state of grasping is said to be "separate." What could this mean? Simply that the experience of craving *intensifies the split between subject and object* (between "me" and "the ice cream"), so that it appears that *without* the object of my grasping I am unwhole. Without the object of my desire I am bereft. Empty. Unfulfilled. Grasping amplifies the sense of separation from the object. Indeed, grasping splits the world between subject and object—heightening the intensity of wanting so that it proliferates into an ever-increasing cycle of wanting and getting and then wanting again—and more. In this state, the mind can never feel whole. It is damned to an eternal sense of separation and emptiness.

So: Disturbed. Obscured. Separate.

Krishna has captured these very insights in his teaching to Arjuna: "When you keep thinking about sense objects," he says, "attachment comes. Attachment breeds desire, the lust of possession that burns to anger. Anger clouds the judgment; you can no longer learn from past mistakes. Lost is the power to choose between what is wise and what is unwise, and your life is utter waste."

Lost is the power to choose between what is wise and what is unwise.

These states of craving for what we might call "gross objects of desire" are easy to see everywhere in our daily life. Simply pay attention. You'll see them hour by hour in your own life as they manifest in grasping for food, for sex, for pleasure, for comfort. What is not so easy to see are the ways in which grasping colors our motivation toward more subtle objects of desire—in our work, in our play, even in our spiritual life. We can just as easily get caught up in craving while we're sitting in meditation, or doing yoga. We can crave exalted states. Enlightenment. We can crave exalted performance even in our most sublime dharma work. Grasping exerts its pernicious effects even in the most refined areas of human endeavor. And wherever it shows up, yogis rightly found that it creates suffering, and that it *has a disabling effect on performance.*

What is the antidote? Krishna counsels "detachment." "Seek refuge in the attitude of detachment," he teaches, "and you will amass the wealth of spiritual awareness." But here is an important proviso: not detachment from the passionate involvement in the task at hand; not detachment from one's dharma. Detachment from the outcome.

"Neither agitated by grief nor hankering after pleasure, [the yogis] live free from lust and fear and anger . . . Fettered no more by selfish attachments, they are neither elated by good fortune nor depressed by bad."

Krishna makes here an important link. When the mind is not colored by grasping it is free—free of disturbance, obscuration, and separation. The mind is at ease. It is seeing clearly. And it is in union with all beings. Nonseparate! And when the mind is in this excellent and most refined state we are free to truly absorb ourselves in dharma. When there is no obsessive concern with outcome, with gain of any kind, we are able to become completely absorbed in what we're doing—our actions and thoughts undivided by worry. All of our energy can become concentrated on the task at hand.

"When consciousness is unified," says Krishna, "all vain anxiety is left behind. There is no cause for worry, whether things go well or ill."

All vain anxiety is left behind! These are moments of peace, and possibility. "When you move amidst the world of sense, free from attachment, and aversion alike, there comes the peace in which all sorrows end, and you live in the wisdom of the Self."

— 2 —

This all sounds wonderful. Heaven on earth. But how in God's name do we accomplish this feat? How do we rid ourselves of desire? For desire seems woven into the very fabric of human life.

Arjuna—rightly distrustful of this teaching—will ask the very questions we want to ask: Isn't it precisely desire that motivates action? Isn't it our very desire for success and for achievement—and even, indeed, for dharma—that pushes us forward toward the noble things in life? Isn't desire, in fact, a central aspect of our very humanity?

This is where the rubber meets the road. We cannot make any forward movement in our practice of detachment until we understand Krishna's response to this central question. Krishna does not disappoint: He makes a brilliant response, and one that is backed up by centuries of yogic investigation into the pitfalls and possibilities of desire. Krishna's response to these concerns is certainly the most innovative and revolutionary aspect of the Bhagavad Gita. In order to fully appreciate the revolutionary quality of his response, we need a little background.

Even the earliest yogis—going back at least to the ninth century BCE—had begun to understand the pernicious effects of grasping. And they wrestled with a number of strategies to attenuate its power. The first strategy they used was a caveman strategy for dealing with the problem. Eradicate desire. Kill it! Wipe it out. Club it to death. In the early centuries of the yoga tradition, practitioners investigated extreme forms of asceticism as an antidote to grasping. Kill all desire. Root it out. This caveman strategy had a serious flaw. Along with grasping, it also tended to kill all that was good in the practitioner—and not infrequently it actually killed the practitioner himself.

Yogis had to go back to the drawing board on this one. They investigated the problem more deeply. In deep states of meditation, they investigated these very states of desire. Of what were these states composed? As a result of this skillful meditative practice, they began to see more deeply into desire. They found that desire is actually a compound state. It is made up, in part, of grasping and craving, which always and everywhere lead to the experience of suffering. But there are other components of desire as well. There are *salutary* aspects to desire. They discovered an energy at the heart of desire that is full of aspiration for the most noble qualities of the human being. They discovered, too, that allied with these aspirations are profound energies of "resolve" and "strong determination" to achieve the good and the noble. There were components of this state of desire that seemed to come from the highest nature of a human being.

They called these salutary components of desire "aspiration." Aspiration does not have the coloring of afflicted states. There is no *disturbance* in aspiration; rather there is a state of inner calm abiding, and quiet determination. There is no *obscuration* in aspiration; rather what arises is a capacity to see clearly. There is no *separation* in states of aspiration; rather, what emerges are profound states of union with all beings. Aspiration, as it turns out, is full of energy. Full of resolve. Full of a deep ardency for the realization of the Self. It is this very aspiration that leads us to search for truth. For beauty. For our full humanity.

Would it be possible, then, to harness these deeper, more ardent aspects of desire—and at the same time to skillfully pare away its *afflicted* aspects? Could these different components of desire—grasping and aspiration—actually be teased apart?

This teasing apart is at the very heart of the genius of the Bhagavad Gita. The authors of the Gita presented an entirely new strategy. The practitioner can, in fact, tease grasping apart from aspiration, by *harnessing desire to dharma*. And so, we have Krishna's first three teachings: Find your dharma. Do it full out! Let go of the outcome. This frees the natural passion of the human being to be put in the service of dharma. This is the way to live a passionate life without being caught in the fetters of grasping. Do your work passionately. Then let go. Now you are free.

My experience is that the teasing apart of grasping and aspiration is the work of a lifetime. It is slippery. Grasping can often masquerade as aspiration. Aspiration itself can be confused for grasping. The stories that follow in Part IV will explore the ways in which this complex process shows up in real lives—and they will help us investigate three important principles:

1. Let desire give birth to aspiration.
2. When difficulties arise, see them as your dharma.
3. Turn the wound into light.

In Chapter Eight, we will look at the brief but fantastic life of John Keats—one of the greatest poets in the English language, whose life was a bonfire of desire for dharma. We can see in his life the precise ways in which desire, when treated skillfully, inexorably does give birth to aspiration. In Chapter Nine, we will examine a chapter in the life of the great Jungian analyst Marion Woodman—a prolific writer and teacher, author of more than twenty books on Jungian analysis. We will look particularly at the problems that arise when aspiration founders on the shoals of difficulty. And we will see how difficulty itself can be a profound healer. And finally, we'll look at the very, very afflicted life of Ludwig van Beethoven, who skillfully used his burning desire for his dharma to light up not only his own life of suffering, but the life of the whole world.

EIGHT

John Keats:
Let Desire Give Birth to Aspiration

Mark was my best friend in college. The only friend, really, who remained a constant presence in my life long after graduation day. We were close right up to the time of his tragic death at the age of forty-four.

Mark and I didn't really "get" each other until sophomore year, when he lived across the hall from me in an ancient, battle-scarred dorm at the center of the Amherst College campus. I say we didn't "get" each other right away. In fact, as a freshman, Mark scared me. He was a kind of campus celebrity—charming, skillfully extroverted, handsome, and (at least I imagined, and he later denied) popular with the whole cross-section of Amherst society—from jocks to intellectuals. Remember: I had just trucked in from the cornfields of Ohio, and I was awed by the tony (and still all-male) world of Amherst College. I was much less well prepared—both socially and intellectually—than all those boys who had been to elite New England prep schools. I spent most of my waking time trying to just fit in. Mark didn't have to try. He *was* in. He occupied center stage naturally and without pretense.

The headline of Mark's obituary in *The New York Times* read, "Mark Stevenson, Actor." But I always thought it should have said poet. He was a poet at heart. He dressed like a poet. Spoke like a poet. In fact, before we became friends I had heard around campus that Mark identified with the poet John Keats—and later, when we became close, he sometimes mused with me about his hunch that he might actually be a reincarnation of Keats. How exotic.

But who *was* John Keats, anyway, I thought. And who were these guys who at eighteen years of age were already so knee-deep in life that they could identify themselves with such a luminary? Of course, I had no idea who *I* was, or who I wanted to be. I tended to corral myself with the other freshmen who were also obviously at sea in this elite new world, and were quietly crying homesick tears into their pillows at night. (I could sniff out these boys: that deer-in-the-headlights look. This was my tribe in freshman year.)

It took me the whole of freshman year to stop holding my breath. When I arrived back at Amherst for sophomore year, everything looked different. I had had a construction job all summer. I had—miraculously—added almost an inch and a half of height since my first day at Amherst a year earlier. I was muscled and tan. I'll never forget driving onto campus that fall. Amherst looked for the first time like a place I could call home. I was not going to just survive this year, I said to myself. I was going to thrive. And as I settled into my dorm room, there was Mark Stevenson—rooming right across the hall from me. My luck had turned. Mark and I became friends that very day. And throughout the fall, we got into the habit of taking long walks in the New England woods surrounding the village. We hiked the nearby Holyoke Range together. By late October we were sitting at the top of Memorial Hill late into the night, sharing our adolescent secrets.

I continued to watch Mark in awe. But now I watched him up close. I watched throughout the next three years, as he went on being more and more himself—passionate about his many pursuits, and not particularly caring what others thought of him. At some point—after he had pledged one of the most elite fraternities—he decided, apparently, to *live* like the John Keats he thought he might be. He decorated his room like that of an eighteenth-century lord, complete with suits of armor and tapestries (where on earth did he find them?). He called me Cope, as if we were scholars at Oxford. He created around him an aura of another world. To live with Mark was to live inside a great drama.

— 2 —

There are aspects of our lives that we can never fully understand without the perspective of age. When I was a graduate student, studying psychoanalytic psychotherapy, a mentor of mine said, "Psychoanalysis is to help the patient acknowledge, experience, and bear reality." Yes, I thought. This made sense. But then he added a line that I did not really understand at the time: "And to put it all into perspective." *Acknowledge, experience, and bear reality. And put it into perspective.* Much of the developmental work of middle and old age is precisely about putting experience into perspective—about understanding perhaps for the first time what one's life really means.

Mark's story has only come into perspective for me deep into middle age. In fact, I don't think I ever fully appreciated Mark until I began to study the life of John Keats. As much as Mark had tried to educate me about Keats (oh, all that poetry he read aloud at night in our dorm room, and quoted by heart on our walks on the Holyoke Range), I never really *got it.* I realize now that one cannot understand Mark—or anyone— without understanding his exemplars, his mentors, his heroes.

In the last ten years, I have indulged a fascination with Keats. And, strangely perhaps, this has happened in large part as a result of my interest in the Bhagavad Gita. When I started studying the Gita, I just couldn't get Keats out of my mind. Vague memories from college began to haunt me. And then I realized: *Keats was a man who was in love with his dharma.* The idea of dharma was the key to understanding Keats's life!

At the age of eighteen, in 1813, John Keats discovered what he called his "vocation to poetry." Keats—celebrating the miracle of finding his calling—wrote in an early attempt at a long poem, "O, for ten years, that I may overwhelm Myself in poesy; so I may do the deed That my own soul has to itself decreed." I began to understand Mark's fascination with this guy.

From the first moments of the discovery of his dharma, John Keats was aware of a willingness to let himself be "used" by his calling. "The genius of poetry," he said at the tender age of nineteen, "must work out its own salvation in a man." (Who understands these things at the age of nineteen?) Within six years of trying his hand at poetry, Keats would have written some of the most brilliant verse in the English language. Soon after that he would be dead.

Keats was living his dharma, to be sure. But it gets even more exciting than that. He independently discovered—out of necessity—the pillars of The Doctrine of Inaction in Action. He was *letting himself be used by his dharma.* He had stumbled onto the secret of "not the Doer" (a central principle of dharma that we will explore later on). In his very short but intense life, Keats had intuited many of the most central teachings of the Gita, and had put them to work for himself. His greatness is based on these very discoveries.

As I dug into Keats's life, Mark's story, too, began to haunt me. After graduate school, Mark had gone on to write a one-man play about Keats, entitled *This Living Hand: A Visitation from John Keats,* which he performed for many years in New York and around the United States and Europe. I wondered how deeply Mark himself—through his association with Keats   had wandered into dharma territory. Perhaps he, too, had really understood The Doctrine of Inaction in Action. This was an exciting thought for me: Perspective can at times bring exhilaration.

I rummaged around in my photo albums, and pulled out pictures of Mark—not only from college, but also from our many adventures together during our thirties and forties. I found a photo of Mark standing on a mammoth rock jutting out into the ocean in northern Rhode Island, taken while we were on a summer bicycling trip. His head is tossed back, his shoulder-length blond hair blowing in the ocean breeze. I hung the picture over my writing desk.

And then I realized it for the first time: Mark looked remarkably like Keats. I mean—astonishingly. Both were short of stature and compact—handsome, blond, with beautiful smiles and chiseled features. How could I have missed this? Joseph Severn, one of Keats's closest friends, had once described Keats as seeming taller than his true height because of his erect bearing, and a "characteristic backward toss of the head." I looked again at the picture: There it was in Mark. The backward toss of the head. Severn also described "a particularly dauntless expression, such as may be seen on the face of some seamen." Mark, again. Reincarnation? Really?

Having gone this far, I knew that I had to know everything about

Keats's journey. I dug into biographies and collections of his poetry in search of his dharma story.

It's easy to be put off while reading about great lives. We tend to read them backward, and inevitably to gild them in the process. We read Keats through the prism of his fame, his final few poems. But what happens if you read Keats's life forward—the way it actually unfolded?

Read this way, Keats is a much more interesting character. He's courageous. He's tragic. He died at twenty-five—penniless and almost entirely alone in a foreign land—of a ravaging and wasting disease. He and his work were mostly unknown when he died. By the time of his death, he had published only a few slim volumes of poetry—much of which was really not that good—but some of which was the most phenomenal and daring verse yet to be written in English.

Keats and his friends and associates alike all assumed he had died without realizing his potential. And yet. Read his story, and you will see that he *did* bring forth what was within him. Not in great volumes, but in marvelous intensity. Poetry had, finally, saved John Keats. Just as the Civil War had saved Walt Whitman. Just as painting landscapes had saved Camille Corot. And did Mark's writing save him?—I wondered as I sniffed out Keats.

Keats did not achieve fame until many decades after his death. Indeed, it would be a century after his death before his reputation was really established. I don't expect Mark to achieve fame—or at least any more than he already has. But that is not the point. Did Mark, in his short life, have a fulfilling experience of bringing forth what was within him? Did Keats's lessons help Mark live an exuberantly full life? Had Mark already learned—through Keats—what I am only learning now? And had Mark actually tried to share with me, even as an undergraduate, his excitement about dharma?

—— 3 ——

After studying Keats's life closely for many years, Keats's biographer, Aileen Ward, concluded that "He was not one of those rare poets who are born, not made. He lacked the endowments or opportunities with which the other great poets of his time started . . . He was to rise above his own narrow background by stubborn ambition and hard work, making himself a poet by studying the best examples of poetry he could find and absorbing what he could from them."

Stubborn ambition and hard work. Just like the rest of us. *Not a genius.* A product, rather, of deliberate practice. Keats's story is one of strong determination. It is a story of desire for the realization of dharma. And, most important for our purposes now, it is the story of the transmutation of this desire into aspiration, of the transmutation of desire into determined action, and finally into realization. Keats's self-realization required effort, yes—but a particular kind of effort. Precisely the kind that Krishna prescribes to Arjuna: "Do your dharma passionately, but let go of the fruits." This is, for me, where the story of Keats's life becomes truly exemplary.

—— 4 ——

John Keats was born in London to a working-class family. He had an apparently happy childhood. But disaster struck in his early teens. His father died in a riding accident at the slim age of thirty, and his mother died not long afterward at age thirty-six—when Keats was only fourteen—succumbing to what Keats would later call the "family disease"—tuberculosis.

Much of Keats's poetry seems to have been an attempt to work through the almost unbearable losses of his early life. From its rough beginnings, his poetry is saturated with a sense of the fragility of life and love—and the transience of beauty. He wrote repeatedly about

Beauty that must die,
and joy, whose hand is ever at his lips
Bidding adieu; and aching Pleasure nigh
turning to poison while the bee-mouth sips.

A quality of "paradise lost" saturates much of Keats's greatest poetry. In his work—as in his life—beauty and happiness appear as unearthly visitors, inevitably evaporating as quickly as they came, leaving him bereft on the empty shores of life.

From childhood onward throughout his short life, Keats had to grapple with the realities of impermanence—the realities so often emphasized by Krishna in his long talks with Arjuna. Keats discovered early on that he could hold on to nothing. And so his *koan*—the central question of his life—became how to live life fully without holding on to it. How to *have* it without possessing it. "Kiss the joy as it flies," says William Blake. In order to become a great poet, Keats would have to work through the *problem of grasping*. The evidence that he finally did learn to live in the stream of impermanence is written—at his instruction—on his very tombstone: "Here lies one whose name was writ in water."

Precisely how Keats used poetry to work through this great existential problem—the problem of grasping—is for me an endlessly compelling story. He worked it all out through words.

As I have said, Keats's mother died a gruesome death when he was only fourteen. This appalling event turned young Keats into a voracious reader. Through books he absorbed himself in the world of great men and daring deeds—the worlds of Julius Caesar and Brutus and of William Tell and William Wallace. Early on, one can see Keats's attempts to master his difficult circumstances through *imagination*. Even at the age of fourteen he was beginning to gather together the skills of the poet. ("Poetry," Cyril Connolly has said, "comes from the ferment of an unhappy childhood working through a noble imagination.")

Soon, into his fifteen-year-old life, came the next essential ingredient of a great poet: a mentor. Keats's world was vastly expanded when he met the most important friend of his youth: Charles Cowden Clarke. Clarke, just eight years older than Keats, was the son of the headmaster of Keats's school, and he was an extraordinarily bright and generous friend to Keats. Clarke noticed that Keats seemed to devour books rather than read them, and he took an interest in this handsome, lively, and engaged boy. He introduced Keats to Chaucer and Shakespeare and Spenser, and challenged him in vigorous debate about the issues of the day.

Keats responded well to Clarke's interest. His imagination and intellect came alive. The stories of their friendship—later told by Clarke—are compelling. At the drop of a hat, the two friends would walk the fifteen miles to London to see their favorite actor, John Kemble, on stage in Shakespeare's plays, and then walk back, arriving home at dawn, having talked through the entire night.

Keats was a sensitive boy, and particularly sensitive to beauty. Clarke helped wake in him a latent love of nature, during what would become long, thoughtful walks in the countryside around the school. English poets, it seems, are forever walking. From Wordsworth to Auden. And as I read the stories of Keats becoming a walker, I could not but think of my walks with Mark in the hills around Amherst. We walked constantly, vigorously, in all seasons, but almost always talking as we went, about literature, music, art, love, life's vicissitudes.

— 5 —

Keats had little interest in poetry until he was almost eighteen. One afternoon, probably in the summer of 1813, Clarke read Edmund Spenser's "Epithalamion" aloud to Keats, and as he was reading, Clarke looked up to see Keats's face positively "alight with pleasure."

The encounter with Spenser's poems was a turning point. That night Keats went home with the first volume of *The Faerie Queene*. The next time they met, Clarke "discovered that he had gone through the book like a young horse through a spring meadow, ramping." By Clarke's account, it was as though Keats had fallen deeply in love—overnight.

The first encounter with dharma is very often described as falling in love. When we see our dharma—smell it, feel it—we *recognize* it. It is chemical. Undeniable. Keats was smitten. At the beginning, he did not have any apparent genius for poetry. Just a love of it. And he knew—in the way that we know these things—that poetry was just the right vessel for him. Clarke introduced Keats to the principles of poetry as they had been held in England for the previous hundred years, and together, Clarke and Keats began to read the standard authors, from Milton to Gray. In his spare time, Keats began to write poetry, though he withheld his early efforts even from his mentor until much later.

—— 6 ——

Keats was, like most of us—like Arjuna—full of doubt about the viability of his dharma. Throughout his teens, he was almost constantly involved in an inner struggle around his identity. In an attempt to develop a practical career, he apprenticed to an apothecary, determined to move toward the medical profession. He felt keenly the need to make his way in the world. He was bright enough to succeed in medicine. And he was determined to do some good for the world. Early on in his apprenticeship, indeed, he did rise to the top of the field, and he was given prized positions among his peers.

But from the start, Keats was conflicted about medicine. In fact, this doctor in training was sickened by the very sight of illness. He had never recovered from seeing his mother's slow death from tuberculosis. As a result, he overidentified with his patients and their suffering. He likely would have been a very unhappy physician.

With the discovery of poetry, Keats's interest in medicine began to wane. He cut classes. And when he did go to class, he sat absorbed in the working out of a poetic image or the structure of a sonnet. Some of his classmates later described him as lazy, as indolent—and as a dreamer. They had no idea what he was working out in his notebooks.

For several years, Keats wrestled intensely with his doubt. His choice was between a mainstream career—with its imagined security, money, and position—and the never-really-acceptable life of the poet. He saw clearly enough that to be a poet is to live on the edge. No security in that life.

By his eighteenth year, Keats had worked through much of his ambivalence: He resolved to become a poet. His desire first showed itself as a burning ambition. He wanted to be, as he said, among the first of the English poets. His ambition at this time was so great that he reportedly told his brothers that if he did not succeed he would kill himself. Keats told his friend Henry Stephens that poetry was "the only thing worthy of the attention of superior minds," and that to rank among the poets was the chief object of his ambition. He threw himself into poetry with the energy almost of despair.

—— 7 ——

Sometime in 1816, when he was about twenty years old, Keats began to intentionally take on the *look* of the poet. He appeared with his neck nearly bare, like the then-fashionable poet Lord Byron. He took to wearing loose trousers like a sailor's and a short seaman's jacket (also Byronic). He let his own thick curls grow long, and experimented with a series of mustaches. Keats was posing as a poet. This is what we do in the early stages of finding our dharma. We try it on. As W. H. Auden noted, "human beings are by nature actors who cannot become something until they have first pretended to be it."

Keats was on fire with his dharma. "I find that I cannot exist without Poetry," he said. "Half the day will not do." His early enthusiasm for dharma is expressed in a long, rambling, and ecstatic poem called "Sleep and Poetry." One night, after a languorous dinner party during which the talk was of nothing but poetry, Keats was too excited to sleep. Lying in bed, he had a waking dream of his own destiny. His vision expanded to a vision of his own future as a poet—and not only that, but to the past of English poetry and his intersection with it. He allowed himself to feel his kinship with Chaucer and Shakespeare and Milton.

This turned out to be a pivotal moment in Keats's dharma story. It marked his discovery of his own artistic lineage—and most important, his connection with William Shakespeare. Just as one cannot really understand Mark without understanding Keats, one cannot understand Keats without knowing Shakespeare. From the days of his romps with Charles Cowden Clarke, Keats had been devoted to the Bard, but now his interest and affinity deepened. He put up a picture of Shakespeare over his writing desk, and it would remain there for the rest of his life. He now found new meaning in line after line of Shakespeare. He reread the plays and the sonnets. He copied out the sonnets and emulated them in his own writing.

This move toward Shakespeare is central in Keats's dharma story. Every one of us who takes his dharma seriously will search for exemplars. On fire with our own dharma, we sniff out others who are working in the same dharma gold mine as we. Jane Goodall sniffed it out in Louis Leakey, her famous mentor. Susan B. Anthony in Charlotte Brontë, whose pictures, as I have said, hung over her bureau until her death. Beethoven, as we will see, found it in Bach.

What role do these exemplars play? We see in them the full expression of a kindred dharma. We see in them the full flower of what we know exists as a *seed* within our own self. These exemplars become essential doorways for us into our own dharma. They become transitional objects. We read them, study them, take them apart and put them back together again, just as Keats did with Shakespeare. We ingest them. And eventually, through them, we are awakened to our own idiosyncratic genius, just as Arjuna is eventually awakened to his dharma through his relationship with his exemplar, Krishna.

We cannot really understand another human being without understanding his dharma story. And we cannot understand his dharma story without grasping the importance of his dharma mentors. The more I dug into Keats, the more I discovered that one cannot understand Keats without understanding Shakespeare. Mark apparently discovered the same thing. His second major play would be about Shakespeare.

— 8 —

Keats's desire to express himself—fueled by his increasing identification with Shakespeare—was now at the flood. It was at this moment that he declared: "O for ten years, that I may overwhelm Myself in poesy;" He feared, of course, that his life would not be long enough to realize his "genius." Remember his history: His father died at thirty, his mother at thirty-six. From his point of view, even a decade seemed a lot to ask.

But Keats now took the next necessary step. He dove headlong into the phase of mastery that we have called *deliberate practice*. His early writing was mediocre. But he discovered that if he persevered, every now and then some truly fine poetry would emerge. It did not come easily. But he found within himself a quality of strong determination that allowed him to persevere. He worked hard. He wrote daily—as he said, always groping for the noble chiseled line.

Keats now entered into his famous competition with English poet Percy Bysshe Shelley, his rival and peer, who had already begun to make a name for himself in poetic circles. Shelley challenged both Keats and himself to write a long narrative poem—of 4,000 lines. The terms of the challenge? The poem must be completed in six months—a formidable task for a young and untried poet.

When Keats decided to commit himself to Shelley's challenge, he had no idea whether he could actually accomplish such a deed. But he decided to bring everything he had to the task. This was his first taste of true "unity in action." He would organize all of his energies in the service of this challenge. In the face of this undertaking, he finally and completely gave up medicine. He did not take the final exam for his apothecary license. This was a key moment, because Keats showed that he was *willing to risk failure.* He was willing to let his dreams of glory die, and actually take on the work—to succeed, or as he said, to be exposed as a fraud.

He realized that there was no way to discover whether he could write a long poem but to try. "I would sooner fail than not be among the greatest," he said. This moment marked the beginning of a shift in Keats's views about fame. He began to see its deleterious effects. "There is no greater sin after the seven deadly than to flatter oneself into an idea of being a great Poet," he wrote to his brother. He realized what he would later call the folly of self-congratulations and lusting after fame—the folly of his early fascination with the laurel crowning.

Keats now headed off to the Isle of Wight, so that he could work uninterruptedly. He spent at least eight hours a day reading and writing. During this period he became for the first time a truly disciplined writer. And he began to examine his writing process—his own motivations and the ecology of his work and energy. He looked critically at his own output. He was writing massive amounts of poetry. But was it good? At one point, during a period of three weeks he wrote well over a thousand lines of poetry, without flagging. And yet, he was not satisfied with the work. He saw that he was writing in the spirit of *cramming.* In the spirit of greed. "A clenched fist was at work," he said.

Keats mentions this insight in a letter to his brother George. "The high idea I have of poetical fame makes me think I see it towering too high above me." He compared it to an attempt to scale the White Cliffs of Dover, and called it "the Cliff of Poesy." He slowly began to see how his own longing and craving for success may have been undermining the quality of his work. Certainly, he saw how his craving for fame and "laurels" created a kind of anxiety that infected his work. ("Those who are motivated only by the fruits of action," teaches Krishna, "are miserable!" *Miserable!* "They are constantly anxious about the results of what they do.")

Keats, in a brilliant intuitive move, now attempted to work out the problem of grasping through the protagonist of the poem he was writing. He has his main character—Endymion—face the *challenge of failure* in his quest. And how does Endymion work it out? He enters what Keats called "the Cave of Quietude," a retreat into the depths of consciousness. In quiet retreat and contemplation, Endymion realizes that success and failure are not the measure of life. He sees the way in which both light and shade, success and failure, and praise and blame, are all parts of life. He sees, even, the ways in which beauty can be revealed through sorrow, and through life's losses. He decides to choose complete surrender to the endless richness of the moment, whatever the moment brings. He decides to embrace both sides of life—the light and the shadow. This was a pivotal moment in the development of Keats's creative consciousness.

—— 9 ——

Keats finished *Endymion* at the age of twenty-one, on November 28, 1817. It was a triumph for the young poet. Not because it was a great poem. It was not. But because of what it had taught him. Keats would later say, famously, that life is the "vale of Soul-making" and his experience of *Endymion* was a soul-maker for him. *Endymion* made Keats a poet, for he realized that real fulfillment was not about the approbation of critics, but rather came naturally through the experience of bringing forth the best that was in him. It was not the poem's success or failure in the eyes of others that created fulfillment for the poet.

Endymion—this one poem—represents almost half of the poetry Keats published in his short lifetime. Its writing occupied him through nearly one-quarter of his poetic career. And it was not, as I have said, an outward success. But it was an *inward success.* He realized that his *having written it* mattered more than *what he had written.* It was the process of bringing everything he had to the table that transformed him.

In the process of his deliberate practice, Keats had had moments of exhilaration. At regular moments during his work, he had experienced a surrender to some greater power. He would later say, "That which is creative must create itself." He discovered, as all great artists do, that there was something *impersonal* at work. Something at work that was *not him*. And to surrender to this larger force gave him a new kind of freedom, and a new sense of faith in the process itself.

He realized (just as Krishna taught Arjuna) that *he was not the Doer. That which is creative must create itself.* Mastery of his art required humility and a capacity for surrender—a receptivity to experience, and to sorrow as well as joy. Having tasted this himself, he saw that this was the very essence of Shakespeare's greatness. (And after *Endymion* his sense of oneness with Shakespeare increased.) He saw that the "immortality" that is gained in the creation of great art is not immortality in anyone else's eyes, but a transcendence of time through the outpouring of the soul's possibility. Indeed, he discovered, as did Shakespeare, that throwing oneself passionately into work brings a changed relationship with time. This was true immortality.

—— 10 ——

With this came a first glimpse, for Keats, of a sublime truth. He realized that the most precious fruit of his art would be the way it allowed him access to the *innermost character of a person or thing*. He saw that poetry was merely a vehicle—a way to *know* the world. A way to know the soul of a person, a landscape, or any object of beauty. He realized that he did not need to *possess* any of it. He only needed to *know* it. And this knowing was what brought not just happiness, but bliss, rapture, and authentic fulfillment.

The question he had been asking—"Wherein lies happiness?"—now had its best answer. "A fellowship with essence!!!" he would exclaim. With this insight, Keats had solved the central riddle of his life: how to have a full experience of life without possessing it—without owning it, without grasping it, without holding on to it.

Hard upon the heels of this discovery came another: Grasping for an object actually interferes with *knowing* it. The discovery that holding on too tightly disturbs the mind, and finally interferes with the mind's capacity to know. This is, of course, the very insight that Krishna teaches to Arjuna.

And so emerged the insight for which Keats is best known by generations of college students: his theory of Negative Capability. He had this remarkable insight on a walk—his favorite time for reflecting—and wrote it down later in a letter to his brother: "Several things dovetailed in my mind," he wrote excitedly to his brother George, "and at once it struck me what quality went to form a Man of Achievement especially in Literature and which Shakespeare possessed so enormously—I mean Negative Capability, that is when man is capable of being in uncertainties, Mysteries, doubts, without any irritable reaching after fact and reason." This Negative Capability also seems to require the capacity for surrender, and the capacity, as Keats said, to "annul the self."

Keats found these insights exhilarating—freeing. "Let us open our leaves like a flower and be passive and receptive—sap will be given us for Meat and dew for drink—I was led into these thoughts . . . by the beauty of the morning operating on a sense of Idleness . . ."

Keats's poetic consciousness now began to move beyond what the contemplative traditions often call the pairs of opposites: gain and loss, praise and blame, fame and ill-repute. He saw how the poet must be open to all experience, light and dark. He saw the importance of leisure, as Frost did. And he began to learn to wait patiently for a gradual ripening.

Observes Aileen Ward: "A year or two earlier he had described the writing of poetry in terms of a journey, a battle, a cliff to be scaled. Now he saw it in images of grain ripening, of wine aging, of the sun rising and setting, the flower which must drink the nature of the soil before it can put forth its blossoming."

Keats now began to formulate his description of the greatest poetic virtue—what he would come to call "disinterestedness." "To bear all naked truths, and to envisage circumstance, all calm," he wrote in "Hyperion." "That is the top of sovereignty." Keats had rediscovered the soul of Krishna's teaching.

In his attempt to put all of this into words, John Keats wrote two sonnets on fame. In the first, he states that fame comes only to the man who has learned to be indifferent to it. In the second, he calls fame "a fierce miscreed" of salvation, and he turns away from his earlier feverish grasping for success toward less aggressive images of unforced growth—toward the gradual unfolding of life that he now perceives to be in the natural order of things. He begins to use images of ripening. "If Poetry comes not as naturally as the Leaves to a tree," he wrote, "it had better not come at all."

—— 11 ——

Now Keats's most mature poetry pours forth. This outpouring must remind us of Thoreau at Walden, after he let go of his grasping for fame and success. Keats, quite aware of his own transformation, writes about it with uncharacteristic understatement: "I think a little change has taken place in my intellect lately."

Keats declared that he would henceforth write "not for Fame and Laurel, but from the mere yearning and fondness I have for the beautiful even if my night's labours should be burnt every morning and no eye ever shine upon them." Ward captures the moment perfectly: "Being a poet, he now realized, was no glorious thing in itself but merely *a fact of his own nature*. What alone mattered was the activity of writing, the kingdom of his own creation which he entered every time he sat down to work. Beside this solitary delight the world's applause or contempt meant nothing."

—— 12 ——

This far into Keats's story, I was stunned by the growing realization that even as an undergraduate Mark Stevenson had fully understood the meaning of Keats's transformation. I remembered, in fact, that Mark had struggled to communicate all of this to me—in those long talks on Memorial Hill, and later as we walked in the woods near my house in Boston. He had tried to tell me about Negative Capability. He had tried to tell me how strangely close he felt to Keats—and later to Shakespeare.

He had tried to tell me how he felt a call to communicate Keats's truth to the current generation, and how lonely it was to have a vocation so few understood or valued.

As I gazed at Mark's picture over my writing desk one morning—with all of these thoughts swirling—I had an idea: Call his mother. Call Dorothy! I hadn't spoken with her since he died—sixteen years earlier. I dialed the number in my old address book. To my astonishment, she picked up the phone. There she was! She must be well into her eighties, I thought. But she sounded well, and completely on top of things as always.

Dorothy caught me up: Her husband, Robert, had died. She had sold the family home and now lived in an assisted-care community. We talked about Mark. About his play. About his last, difficult year. I told her about the book I was writing, about my rediscovery of the meaning of Mark's work, and about the Bhagavad Gita.

I asked Dorothy if she had a copy of the manuscript of *This Living Hand.*

"Yes! I'm pretty sure I've got it packed away somewhere. I'll find it for you."

A week later, there it was on my doorstep with the mail. It was the original manuscript of *This Living Hand,* typed out on a manual typewriter in the early 1970s, with copious cross-outs and notes written in Mark's elegant hand. It all came rushing back.

Dorothy gave me the phone number of her eldest surviving son, John, and I called him as well. We talked at length about Mark. What was Mark's relationship to Keats? What about this old notion that Mark was a reincarnation of Keats? John had clearly thought about these issues.

"We often spoke about his feelings regarding this possibility [of reincarnation]," John wrote to me after our chat. "I do remember a distinct time when he wrestled with this notion, a restless period that ended with his acceptance of what he called 'the spirit of Keats.' This point is supported by two clear examples from Mark's life. First, he told me of his experiences in feeling—and once seeing—Keats's spirit at his house in England and also at his grave in Rome. Neither experience frightened Mark, but rather gave him a sense of calm and joy to be alive and carrying out his dreams of finishing the play and working to improve each scene—much like Keats's own dedication to his poetry. In either case, what happened to Mark was much more than an inspiring moment; I think these occurrences had a lasting effect, and became part of the mysticism of Mark's life forward. He was never afraid of these experiences; they gave him comfort, like meeting up with a long-lost friend who returned for a brief visit."

I had never thought of Mark as a mystic. At no time during our years of friendship did we have that word in our vocabulary. But, of course, it does describe him.

John's letter, too, reminded me of the years, after Mark finished graduate school in Texas, when he was working on *This Living Hand*. I saw now that these were his years of deliberate practice. He wrote and rewrote the scenes. He worked on the dialogue with a coach. He put it through many trial runs in front of live audiences, and then went through weeks or months of driven rewriting. The play went through countless iterations—and I really think that Mark was revising and improving it until he died.

In an attempt to befriend the spirit of John Keats, Mark frequently traveled to England and Rome, to walk in the places where Keats had walked. I realized that these were all part of Mark's efforts to *know* the object of his work—what Keats himself would call "knowing the essence." There must have been fulfillment for Mark in this process. It's clear to me now that Mark absorbed himself in the life and mind of this great poet—until Mark himself disappeared.

I remembered that I had actually witnessed this absorption—this disappearance—when watching his play. John had seen the same thing, and wrote about it in his letter. "I got to see Mark on stage performing *This Living Hand* twice during his college/school tours through Michigan and Ohio," he wrote. "On both occasions I witnessed the character transformation—from my brother Mark to the person of John Keats. I still wonder at Mark's ability to achieve this early in the show and sustain the show by being Keats—not performing as an actor. That ability, that presence, made the show what it was and no other actor could accomplish the same outcome with Mark's play."

It made me happy to hear John say this. Mark had indeed been fully engaged in the work of the poet, the playwright. He had mastered the skills required to produce this magical transformation. And I knew that this mastery itself must have brought him a sense of fulfillment. It was his dharma. He was pursuing it with everything he had.

Twenty years after his death, I understood for the first time the sacrifice that Mark had made for his art. I grasped the meaning of those years of waiting tables and living in a tiny Manhattan apartment. It all made sense, though Mark himself wrestled with his doubts about this sacrifice from time to time. He talked about inevitable comparisons between the trajectory of his life and that of his many Amherst peers who went on to more mainstream lives—and the rewards of money and respectability.

Mark had thought of himself as a vehicle for his work. He found his calling, and dived in utterly. I think, too, that at some point he had really let go of the outcome. He understood that he was not the Doer. Can there be a more exciting life?

— 13 —

At the age of twenty-one, Keats had a premonition of his own death. He came to believe that he had only three more years—"one thousand days," as he said at the time—to realize his gifts.

His premonition was not far off. By the time he was twenty-three, Keats had clearly contracted tuberculosis. All the symptoms were there, and from the Fall of 1818, he continually complained of them: pressure in the chest, coughing, an ever-present sore throat, colds that would not go away, fatigue, and night sweats.

But the shift in consciousness that had taken place through his fierce pursuit of poetry allowed him to face illness and even impending death. He was committed now, "to bear all naked truths, and to envisage circumstance, all calm," he wrote.

Keats began to frame death in an altogether new way. He saw death as "the supreme experience—Life's high meed." While heretofore he had tried to keep out the "disagreeables," he now saw that they had to be fully admitted in. And now, in "admitting in" even death—the great disagreeable—he was expanded and freed.

This reframing of death is his final embrace of "the world as the vale of Soul-making." "Do you not see," he wrote to George, "how necessary a world of pain and troubles is to school an intelligence, and make it a soul? This school is a place where the heart must feel and suffer in a thousand diverse ways!"

—— 14 ——

The final year of Keats's life is often written about as a miracle of creativity. But it is really no miracle. It is only the natural fruition of the process of transformation in which Keats had already been engaged for many years. In the spring of 1818, Keats walked daily on the heath with the now-famous young beauty Fanny Brawne—with whom he was passionately in love. During these months—months almost lifted from time—Keats's most astonishing poetry poured forth. These were the months during which he wrote the so-called "Four Odes of May"—*On Indolence, On a Grecian Urn, To a Nightingale,* and *On Melancholy*—which would forever seal his reputation. In these odes Keats reached his own ripeness as a poet. "For these few weeks," says Ward, "he stood at a point of perfect balance, confident in his ability to meet the future, able to contemplate his past with calm, and rejoicing in the beauty of the season, the joy of an answered love, the delight of a mastered craft—the themes of the odes as well as his incentives to writing them."

During these months of creative exuberance, Keats became an uncharacteristically solitary creature, save for his walks with Fanny. Already sick, and chronically weak and fatigued, he found great relief in quiet, solitary days—days spent writing and studying Italian. He was in love with his work, and fully absorbed in it: "I look upon fine phrases like a lover," he wrote. "Poetry is all I care for, all I live for."

What emerged, finally, in these months lifted from time, was his most astonishing poem: "To Autumn." This is sometimes called the most perfect poem in the English language. Keats called it simply, "Verse that comes not out of the fever of ambition."

To Autumn

Season of mists and mellow fruitfulness,
    Close bosom-friend of the maturing sun;

Conspiring with him how to load and bless
    With fruit the vines that round the thatch-eves run;
To bend with apples the moss'd cottage-trees,
    And fill all fruit with ripeness to the core;
    To swell the gourd, and plump the hazel shells
With a sweet kernel; to set budding more,
    And still more, later flowers for the bees,
    Until they think warm days will never cease,
    For Summer has o'er-brimmed'd their clammy cells.

Who hath not seen thee oft amid thy store?
    Sometimes whoever seeks abroad may find
Thee sitting careless on a granary floor,
    Thy hair soft-lifted by the winnowing wind;
Or on a half-reap'd furrow sound asleep,
    Drows'd with the fume of poppies, while thy hook
    Spares the next swath and all its twined flowers:
And sometimes like a gleaner thou dost keep
    Steady thy laden head across a brook;
    Or by a cider-press, with patient look,
    Thou watchest the last oozings hours by hours.

Where are the songs of Spring? Ay, where are they?
    Think not of them, thou hast thy music too,—
While barred clouds bloom the soft-dying day,
    And touch the stubble-plains with rosy hue:
Then in a wailful choir the small gnats mourn
    Among the river shallows, borne aloft
    Or sinking as the light wind lives or dies;
And full-grown lambs loud bleat from hilly bourn;
    Hedge-crickets sing: and now with treble soft
    The red-breast whistles from a garden-croft;
    And gathering swallows twitter in the skies.

The poem was a quiet triumph. In this poem, Keats's personality is
finally completely out of the way—utterly lost and absorbed in his im-

ages. He has here achieved the effortlessness that Robert Frost describes when he declares that "a poem should ride on its own melting." "To Autumn" was a poem that wrote itself. Creativity creating itself! Keats is now at one with the world.

As it turned out, "To Autumn" was a gesture of farewell. Within months, Keats would be assured of his impending death.

— 15 —

After a bone-chilling coach ride from London (on an outer seat, because the impoverished poet could not afford to sit inside), Keats arrived home seriously ill, flushed and trembling. He climbed the stairs to his room, and as he got into bed a fit of coughing seized him. His friend Charles Brown, who was following him up the stairs with a glass of wine, heard him gasp. Blood was oozing from his lips.

Brown found Keats sitting up in bed, examining the bright red spot on the white sheet. Then, according to Brown's account, Keats looked very steadily up into his friend's face, and said, "I know the colour of that blood. It's arterial blood. There's no mistaking that colour." As calmly as he could, he added, "That blood is my death-warrant. I must die."

— 16 —

In the Fall of 1993, Mark and I went back to Amherst College for Homecoming. I knew that Mark had been sick for some time. But I had never yet really seen him obviously ailing. Now he was clearly ill. He was pale. His face looked strained. He had lost weight.

Still, his mood was exuberant, and he was buoyed by being back at "the fairest college." So I was stunned when, just as we walked onto the campus, he sprinted to a sewer drain in the parking lot and threw up several times—violently. He didn't want to talk about it. We just moved on—walking across the campus, kicking through piles of oak leaves, toward the soccer fields, where we would meet some old friends.

Later that afternoon, Mark and I sat again on Memorial Hill—as the skies turned red with the sunset and the throngs of alums moved toward their dorms to prepare for dinner. I looked closely at Mark. I could see the suffering written on his face. But his exuberance was there as well. There was the regal tilt of the head. The impish grin. Mark was in a mood to reflect on his life. He was glad he had written his plays. They were the chief satisfaction of his life. His many sacrifices for his art had been good and right. "Austen called her books her children," he said. "I know exactly how she felt."

Mark talked about the struggle involved in writing. "I know I'm not a brilliant playwright," he said. "I'm not a natural, really. It didn't come easy. But it was my work to do."

He said, "You know, Keats sometimes wondered about where his poetry came from—marveled at it really. I've felt the same way about my own work so many times." And then he quoted a line from Keats I had not heard: "many a verse from so strange an influence / That we must ever wonder how, and whence It came."

We looked together—and for the last time—out over the expansive view of the Holyoke Range in the distance. Mark talked jokingly about his withering body. He had never really had more than a modest amount of physical vanity. He talked about how Keats had observed the terrifyingly rapid decline of his own body. And Mark reminded me that Keats had become obsessed with the look of his hands as he failed.

It provoked a question. I had never understood why Mark had quoted the whole of Keats's poem "This Living Hand" at the end of his play—or why, in fact, he used that line—out of all the fantastic lines he had to choose from—as his title.

"It was ironic," Mark said. He thought for a moment, looking out at the mountains in the distance. Mark spoke deliberately as he finished his thought. "Keats always had the sense that his greatest poems came from somewhere beyond him. That he was just the channel for them. And his life's work was to prepare himself to channel these poems. At the end, of course, he was full of despair that he had not fulfilled his destiny. His hand was withering. And yet 'this living hand' had written some of the finest poetry in the English language. This living hand, though dying, was now immortal. Through his art, he had conquered time."

NINE

Marion Woodman: When Difficulties Arise, See Them as Dharma

In the several years leading up to his eightieth birthday, my father—unbelievably, impossibly—developed Alzheimer's disease. Its onset was rapid, and within a few years he was completely disabled. Well, not just disabled. Gone. Poof. My handsome and charming father—a college president, admired for his wit, impeccably groomed and dressed, affable, commanding—now sitting blankly in a wheelchair looking into vague space, surrounded by other wheelchaired beings in the same disastrous straits.

Here was an energetic man in his late seventies, still vital, who had decidedly found his dharma early in life and had been living it mightily—until he began the long good-bye of Alzheimer's. It was an unending nightmare for those of us who loved him. I was working on another book at that time—also on dharma—and I wondered as Dad's Alzheimer's rapidly progressed: What was his dharma now?

Dad had been born to a poor family in an Ohio River industrial town. He was a short, skinny kid who'd fought his way to high school every day along a route infested with river-town bullies. He won a scholarship to college—then to graduate school. Education lifted him into a life of meaning. And so he fell in love with the power of learning. He became, as he proudly said, "an educator." This was his dharma. He began his career as a professor of history. Then a dean. Then a college president. He loved his students. Loved his faculty. The guy was lit up. He had plans.

And then: Alzheimer's. Dad's story, of course, is not the least bit unusual. One day we're cooking along nicely with our dharma, with the work of our lifetime. And then, *wham!* Life knocks it all to Hell. Illness. Natural disasters. Divorce. A friend of mine was well-launched in his career as a concert pianist when an automobile accident destroyed his hand. He was driving himself into New York City for a concert. He reached over to get a bottle of water on the passenger seat, and when he looked up—*bam!* His career was over. Walt Whitman had completed *Leaves of Grass* and was on the way to literary gianthood when the Civil War blew the country apart. Nobody cared much about poetry for a long while. Keats had barely launched himself on his brilliant career when he contracted tuberculosis and died.

Difficulties arise. Some small. Some large enough to blow our boats out of the water. That's life. But back to our question: What was Dad's dharma now? He could no longer teach, or even read a book. What would his work be henceforth? What would Krishna say about Dad's dilemma?

Of course, you already know the answer. You've read the title of this chapter. *When difficulties arise, see them as dharma.* Your dharma is the work that is called forth from you at this moment. And like everything in this impermanent world, the work of the moment can change on a dime. Alzheimer's was Dad's new dharma.

—— 2 ——

Most of us do not much like change. We get our mitts around the dharma of the moment, and don't want to let go. Our friend Katherine hung on to her deanship for years, her hands tightly wrapped around the rope as it was painfully pulled through them. Whitman hung on to *Leaves of Grass* for almost a decade—living in the fading glow of his success. Hanging on is our first strategy.

I'll tell you later on in this chapter how Dad managed his hanging-on challenge. It was pretty magnificent. (In fact, he didn't hang on much at all.) But for now, let's start with Mom. She was a little more prone to hanging on than was Dad.

Here is the story. As you can well imagine, my father's meltdown hugely affected his partner of fifty years. Mom: the beautiful Barbara Crothers Cope. In fact, it pretty much put the torch to *her* dharma as well as to his. And what was her dharma? She was a wife and a mother. She was also a poet and a writer. But more than anything, her dharma was to love Dad and to support his career and his life. She loved being the wife of a college president. She loved being the wife of Robert S. Cope, period. She was in love with him from the time they met in college. They had kids—five of us—and we were great (naturally) but in a funny way we were optional (which is a difficult story for another time). Dad was not in any way optional. He was essential. So, Mom was particularly savoring this time in their lives. We kids had gone on to lives of our own. She and Dad traveled together. She joined him in his consulting work abroad, and they had many adventures. We saw the pictures. Mom and Dad in Europe. Mom and Dad in the Philippines. Mom sang as she washed the dishes in the evening.

And then: Alzheimer's. Mom's immediate instinct for dealing with the meltdown of her life was one we will all recognize: She declared war on it. "We're going to fight this thing. We'll get the best doctors."

Here was her plan: We will go on as usual. We will keep things as normal as possible. We will never say the word Alzheimer's. "Your father is who he always was," she said to me, "only slightly diminished. We've got him on the best medications." Mom held on as best she could, holding tight to old patterns. She sat—resolute—in the passenger seat of the car with him as he drove forgetfully, straight through stop signs and red lights.

I do not blame Mom one whit for the strategy she employed to deal with the meltdown of her life. I understand her instinct to treat it this way. Indeed, it was heroic. As things deteriorated, Mom was monumentally self-sacrificing in her caretaking for Dad—as are so many of the wives who sit by their bed-bound husbands, feeding them meals in small spoonfuls. Like these other wives, she put the ridiculous party hat on his head at his eighty-second birthday party, when he did not know who or where he was. The family smiled, aghast.

In Mom's strategy the illness was seen as an alien intruder—the enemy. This was completely understandable. (In the face of their mutual catastrophe, I felt, really, that Mom was entitled to any strategy that she could hold on to.)

I said nothing. But in the back of my head I knew that there was another possible approach to this disaster. A radical one, yes. An approach that involved walking a razor's edge, yes. But one that might transmute some of their suffering into *possibility*. Here's the other approach: Instead of declaring war on Alzheimer's, embrace it. Take the whole bloody mess as your dharma. Take it as your new calling. Name it. Claim it. Live the experience of Alzheimer's consciously, fully. Talk about it. Investigate it. Look high and low for the meaning in it. Experience it. Open to the possibility—yes, even to the slim possibility—that this ordeal could be some kind of crazy initiation into wisdom.

The *Tao te Ching* says, "If you stay in the center and embrace death with your whole heart, you will endure forever."

Embrace death with your whole heart? I remember the first time I read that line from Lao-tzu's masterpiece. I thought: This is crazy talk. But I knew from the bottom of my heart that it was right.

I actually knew of an Alzheimer's patient who tried this approach. He took Alzheimer's as his dharma. He walked the razor's edge. OK, he was a very adept Buddhist meditator, and so maybe his whole life had been a preparation for this final effort. He belonged to a meditation community out West. He became famous for embracing his ordeal as dharma. His whole community participated in it with him, taking it on step by brutal step. His courage transformed a lot of people. It was a high-wire act of skillfulness and courage.

—— 3 ——

Krishna has something to say about all of this. He has a teaching that sheds some light on what we might call the built-in flaw in Mom's declare-war-on-it strategy. But it's a very tricky teaching, and it's not for everyone. It is, indeed, one of the most complex parts of the Gita.

Here's the deal: Mom declared war on her situation, right? Now, if Krishna were sitting with Mom, he would explore this with her very carefully. What, precisely, was she declaring war *on*? They would talk about it. He would gently prod her to examine what she was feeling—to examine *precisely* what she was feeling.

Mom would resist, of course—being Mom (or really just being a human being). But eventually—like Arjuna—she would relent, and begin to ponder Krishna's questions. (I can see her in my mind's eye—tilting her head slightly. Gazing into the middle distance. Taking the question seriously. What *was* she feeling?) Well, it wasn't just *one* thing that she was feeling. It was a whole mix of thoughts, of feelings, and of sensations. Aversion. Hatred. Resistance. Denial. Horror. Repulsion. Anger. Rage. Betrayal. Loss.

Krishna would ask her to explore these very carefully. And then he'd tell her something interesting about the whole lot of them. First, though, he'd have to get a running start by giving Mom his lesson about grasping. And then he'd reveal to Mom that yogi scientists discovered that grasping has a flip side. It is called aversion. Aversion is also known by its many other names, almost all of which Krishna uses at one point or another in his discourse with Arjuna. They are: hatred, disdain, anger, fear, revulsion, judgment. This was all very familiar emotional territory for Mom. She knew its peaks and valleys.

Krishna would continue. He would teach Mom that grasping and aversion are twins: They are mirror images of each other. They both involve a rejection of *how it is in this moment*. The grasping mind says, "I long for that experience over there. That experience looks very pleasant. Let's go there." The aversive mind, on the other hand, says, "I hate the way it is right now. This is very, very unpleasant. Get me out of here!" The aversive mind pushes away the unpleasant.

Do you see? Mom was stuck in aversion. "This Alzheimer's will not stand. It will be war. I hate this. I reject this. I will fight this to the bloody end."

What's the problem? Well, you won't be surprised to learn that yogis, looking closely at these difficult aversive states, found that aversion has exactly the same deleterious effects on the mind as grasping does. Remember our friends disturbance, obscuration, and separation? Yep. The aversive mind is visited by each of them.

It's not hard to see how this happens. First, aversion *disturbs* the mind. Anyone can see this. Then, aversion *obscures* our capacity to see clearly. This, too, is obvious. When we're hating something, we do not tend to see it clearly. We see the object of our hatred as all bad—not a mixture of bad and good and neutral as it really is. And finally, and probably most painfully, aversive states *separate* us from ourselves and from others. "I hate this moment. Get me out of this moment. I do not want it to be like this." Aversion is a seat in hell. It separates us from *now*. When the mind is colored by aversion, we can never be at ease—can never have a moment's peace.

Aversion is a notoriously slippery creature. It can begin very, very small, with the simple internal act of moving away from the unpleasant. "I don't like the way I'm feeling just now. I think I'll turn on the TV. Maybe that will help distract me." Avoiding the unpleasant: What could be more human? But this simple impulse to move away from the unpleasant can snowball. Krishna details the inevitable movement of aversive states: The impulse to eschew the unpleasant leads to avoidance; avoidance leads to aversion; aversion leads to fear; fear leads to hatred; hatred leads to aggression. Unwittingly, the oh-so-natural instinct to avoid the unpleasant becomes the root of hatred. It leads to war: war within, war without. Entertaining aversion is a slippery slope.

—— 4 ——

So, Mom was caught in the vise of aversion. You might reasonably observe: *Well, of course she was.* Wasn't that perfectly natural? We do not want these experiences of suffering.

Absolutely right. But Krishna will point out a subtle distinction here. Mom's problem was not her aversion to Alzheimer's. That was perfectly natural. It was her *aversion to her own aversion* that was the problem. She *hated* the aversion. She hated the feeling of aversion itself. She hated the fact that she felt it. She was not comfortable with her anger, with her rage, with her disdain. Her proper WASP tool kit did not include the instruction manual for this level of aversion. She was ripped apart by it.

The great Buddhist teacher Chögyam Trungpa Rinpoche called this experience of aversion to the aversion "the pain of pain." Pain is inevitable, of course. And aversion is a natural response to it. But aversion to the aversion? This is not inevitable, as it turns out. This part is optional. And the kicker: The aversion to the aversion is where the *real* suffering lies. As my friend the American Buddhist teacher Sylvia Boorstein says so often: Pain is inevitable. Suffering is optional.

If Mom (in our imagined dialogue between Krishna and her) had finally opened her mind to this teaching, Krishna would have been able to help her quite a bit. He could had helped her with the pain of pain.

Remember Krishna's brilliant approach to working with desire? Go *into* the desire. Feel it. Explore it. Discover what exactly is in that stew of craving, of wanting. Maybe even find magnificent things in it, like aspiration.

OK: *It's exactly the same teaching with aversion.* Go *into* it. Go into your anger, your fear. Feel it in the body. Get to know it. Find the energy at its heart. Find the secret gift at its center. Don't be afraid. Let it wash over you. *Know* it.

All of the Eastern contemplative traditions stumbled onto this brilliant principle: When difficulties arise, give yourself to them.

When difficulties arise, see them as dharma. This does not come naturally to us. Our instinct is to avoid discomfort at every turn. And we live in a culture that helps us to distract ourselves from discomfort's every manifestation. No! counsels Krishna. Do not try to distract yourself! Try it just the other way 'round. Rather, go into the heart of the difficulty. Experience it. Investigate it. Take yourself into the center of the conflict. Learn to tolerate its discomfort without acting or reacting.

And what do you find at the heart of fear, dread, loathing, anger, hatred? You find a surprise. You find a gift.

A gift at the center of hatred? A gift at the center of aversion? Could it possibly be? I am skeptical. Show me just one person who really lives this way—diving into the burning heart of aversion. This would be one person in a million.

Well, our next exemplar is one of those people. Her name is Marion Woodman. She is one of the world's greatest Jungian analysts and teachers. She was squarely in the middle of a brilliant career when she was struck down with a virulent form of cancer. She was told she would die—indeed, that she would die a very painful death. *Wham!* So much for your brilliant career, Marion. So much for your dharma. And what was Marion's dharma to be now?

Marion did the unusual. She decided to take cancer as her new dharma. She walked the razor's edge: She did not declare war on it. She invited it in to see what she could make of it, and to see what it would make of her. She opened to the possibility that this experience could transform her in salutary ways. Marion lived with her husband of many years—Ross Woodman, a distinguished scholar and author. And Ross—heroically—took it on as well. They walked the razor's edge together. And they discovered, eventually, The Gift at the center of cancer.

Stand at the center and embrace death with your whole heart. Then you will endure forever.

—— 5 ——

Marion Woodman is, as I have said, one of the world's best-known Jungian analysts. She is a widely admired author of important books on feminine psychology and on the relationship between the psyche and the body, including such influential works as *Addiction to Perfection, The Owl Was a Baker's Daughter,* and *Leaving My Father's House.* She has become well known for her lively collaborations with American poet Robert Bly, with Rumi scholar Coleman Barks, and with author Thomas Moore and others. She is a member of an illustrious family: Her brothers are the late Canadian actor Bruce Boa and the well-known Jungian analyst Fraser Boa.

Marion and I have been friends for twenty years. We first met in 1994. I called her on the phone one day entirely out of the blue. Knowing her only by reputation, I called her at her office in Toronto to invite her to speak at a conference I was organizing at Kripalu. It was a conference on psychotherapy and spirituality. Marion had a reputation as a spellbinding speaker on the topics of women, feminine psychology, psychotherapy, and spirituality, and I wanted her voice at this conference.

I was moved by our brief phone call. The voice on the other end of the phone was warm but commanding. It was much as I had imagined it might be, but softer, maybe older. "Well, Stephen," Marion said after we had chatted for a while and I had laid out for her the parameters of the conference I wanted her to address, "I must say you have intrigued me. However, I have to tell you that I am not very well just now. I may not even make it to the podium."

I had no idea how literal Marion was being. She was hugely unwell. She was maybe even dying. She didn't say—and I had no way of knowing—that she was deep in the middle of a life-and-death struggle with cancer, and had just finished a wracking series of radiation treatments. In fact, I would not truly understand what had transpired in that phone call until I read about it years later in her book *Bone*—published after she had narrowly survived her struggle. To this day I marvel that that she came to our conference. (She told me later that she was "listening to inner guidance.") I told Marion on the phone that day that I understood she was "not particularly well," and that we would be delighted to have her join us for the conference, and would consider it a bonus if she were able to speak. Just come, Marion, I said.

Well, as it turned out, Marion did come, and she *was* feeling well on the day of the conference. She *was* able to speak. It was an unforgettable moment. Marion approached the podium slowly, regally. I had not yet seen her in person. She was of medium height, with beautifully coiffed graying hair, and warm blue eyes. I imagined her to be in her late fifties. She had a marvelous, chiseled, intelligent face and beautiful skin and eyes—the face of a Shakespearean beauty, I thought, and the poise of a diva. Had she been an actress, I wondered? Marion showed no sign of radiation-induced weakness, though I learned later how devastating the damage was, and how much pain she was actually in.

That day on the podium, she was, as it turned out, right in the middle of taking her cancer on as her dharma. Of embracing it. Of opening to the journey that was cancer.

—— 6 ——

On November 16, 1993, deep into her career as a Jungian analyst, Marion was diagnosed with cancer of the endometrium. "Talked to Dr. Fellows," she writes in her journal on that fateful day. "He made it clear that I have carcinoma of the endometrium, with a three-doctor check. I made it clear to him that I am not 70—that I still have things to do with my life." I have plans, she said. Plans! (This is just what my father would have said to his Alzheimer's doctor if he had been offered the luxury of such a conversation.)

Cancer provoked an immediate crisis in both Marion's personal life and her professional life. It wildly interrupted a perfectly sublime dharma. But Marion realized, overnight, that she had a *new* dharma. It was called cancer. She wrote in her journal: "When [God] is moving you toward a new consciousness, you need to recognize the winds of change at once, move with them instead of clinging to what is already gone." Wow. Not much holding on there. It was an instinctive move: Recognize the winds of change at once. Move with them.

Marion is a woman who is compelled to find meaning in experience. Indeed, the view that all experience has meaning is the very tenet that had drawn her to Carl Jung's work in the first place. Now she insisted on understanding the meaning of her cancer. "I persevered," she said in the preface to *Bone,* "in trying to experience its many shocks as symptoms attempting to bring healing—wholeness into my body-soul connection."

In *Bone,* Marion describes how she saw her illness as "Destiny." (Her view of Destiny is really very similar to our notion of dharma.) "Destiny is recognizing the radiance of the soul that, even when faced with human impossibility, loves all of life." *All of life.* In another journal entry, she writes: "These are strange days, knowing that I have moved into Destiny, knowing I am in exactly the right place, agonizing as it is." No war here whatsoever.

Marion rearranged her life to conform to her new reality. She realized that this process would take every ounce of strength she had. She made careful choices about her time. She began to wind down her analytic practice in Toronto. Over the months to come she would terminate with many of her longtime analysands. She was paring away everything that was not her new dharma. Frost pared his life down to "poet." Susan B. Anthony became a guided missile for the vote. Whitman became a Soldier's Missionary. And Woodman opened her life to the possibilities of cancer.

— 7 —

Marion Woodman has a fascinating dharma story. Until she was fifty years old, she taught English literature and drama at South High School in Toronto. In those years it must have been apparent to anyone paying attention that Marion Woodman was living her dharma. For twenty years, she brought Shakespeare and Keats and Beckett and Dickinson to life for generations of high school students.

During these years, immersed in the world's great literature, she nurtured a world-class mythopoetic consciousness, until finally at midlife she felt a new call—a call to investigate this consciousness more explicitly. At an age when most people are thinking about retirement, Marion packed herself up and headed to Zurich, Switzerland, to train at the Jung Institute.

Marion studied with the top teachers in Zurich. She lived at the zenith of Carl Jung's world. But she told me once that the real initiation into her new dharma came through her own personal analysis with a legendary Jungian analyst in London. In her book *Coming Home to Myself,* she writes about this experience:

In his eighties, he was my analyst.
I had been in England
seeing him for six months,
and was still trying to be efficient.
On Christmas Eve I learned my dog,
who was in Canada, had been killed.
I decided not to waste my evening session
talking about my dog.
I arrived as organized as usual.
At the end, he sat quietly,
then asked me what was wrong.
Nothing, I said, as I put on my coat.
You have not been here, he said.
I told him my dog was dead.
He wept. Wept over my dog.
Asked me how I could waste Christmas Eve

chattering when my soul animal had just died.
Suddenly his weeping made me feel
what I was doing to my soul.
We wept together.
That's when my analysis began.

That's when my analysis began. That's when Marion began what Carl Jung would call the "night sea journey." That's when Marion began pointing her sails into the wind of the unconscious, and made the journey into the parts of herself that had been exiled to the basement and the attic of her body and soul. With the help of her analyst, she made the irrevocable decision to accept whatever she found there.

—— 8 ——

The "night sea journey" is the journey into the parts of ourselves that are split off, disavowed, unknown, unwanted, cast out, and exiled to the various subterranean worlds of consciousness. It is the night sea journey that allows us to free the energy trapped in these cast-off parts—trapped in what Marion would call "the shadow." The goal of this journey is to reunite us with ourselves. Such a homecoming can be surprisingly painful, even brutal. In order to undertake it, we must first agree to *exile nothing.*

Marion taught me that in the process of the night sea journey we expose the shadow. "The shadow is anything we are sure we are not; it is part of us we do not know, sometimes do not want to know, most times do not want to know. We can hardly bear to look," says Marion. "Well," suggests Marion, "do look!!" It will be startling. ("Ourself behind ourself, concealed—should startle most," wrote Emily Dickinson, Woodman's muse.)

"The shadow may carry the best of the life we have not lived," writes Marion. "Go into the basement, the attic, the refuse bin. Find gold there. Find an animal who has not been fed or watered. It is you!! This neglected, exiled animal, hungry for attention, is a part of your self." Marion discovered, of course, that Jung's technique for discovering our exiled parts centered primarily around the analysis of dreams, which Jung called "the royal road to the unconscious."

Marion was endlessly fascinated by the capacity of dream analysis to reunite us with ourselves. And she was fascinated, too, with the structure of dreams. She was astonished to find in dreams the very same dramatic structure she had been teaching in literature and drama. And she came to believe, as Jung did, that at the heart of the unconscious mind there is a panoramic intelligence that is deeply connected with fundamental human consciousness. She came to believe that this was the only true guide for her soul.

After termination with her analyst in London, Marion would henceforth let her life be guided by an ongoing analysis of her own dream world. "Once we know what the dream world is," she writes, "to be without it is to be rudderless. The dream continually corrects our waking course." Marion, like Jung, came to believe that dreams are the path—circular and meandering as it is—to a knowledge of the exiled self.

— 9 —

When Marion finished her training in Switzerland and her analysis in England, she returned to Canada with Ross and set up a psychotherapy practice, using Jungian techniques. Early on, Marion became particularly fascinated with food addictions and eating disorders, because she herself had wrestled with these very issues.

In the early years of her analytic practice, Marion found herself struggling to understand the repetitive themes in the dreams of her addicted clients. This was for her a phase of deliberate practice. She was trying to find patterns in the psyches of her patients—trying to find new paths to healing. She was systematic about it. She says, "I put rows of dreams on the floor of my studio, organized and reorganized them by theme. I marveled at the overwhelming power of the unconscious and at the same time the intensity of its drive toward healing."

Marion discovered an underlying theme in her clients' dreams. She discovered that her addicted clients lived divided lives—lives split between body and soul, between perfection and imperfection, between light and dark. Healing came about through integrating these "pairs of opposites." She came into an understanding of the way in which longing for our idealized images of life separates us from our true selves and from our true callings.

What a relief, then, she discovered, to learn to accept both sides of these pairs of opposites—not just the God in us, but the animal, too. Not just the transcendent states, but the realities of embodied life. "What a relief to be human instead of the god or goddess my parents imagined me to be or I imagined them to be," she declared. She found that her clients experienced the same kind of relief. No matter how painful the truth may be, it's usually a relief to acknowledge it.

— 10 —

Now Marion would use all of her Jungian analytic techniques—especially dream analysis—to come into relationship with cancer. She began a new phase of her dream analysis. Everything became subservient to this work. Marion told me that she would spend hours each morning in bed with her dreams. "A dream not understood is like a letter unopened," wrote Jung. Now these letters—these dreams—were for Marion a matter of life and death.

Her dreams began to teach her about her current state of mind and body. In her dreams, she became aware of feeling trapped. She sensed that light could not penetrate the darkness of her body. "My dark images are related to depression as surely as my cancer is related to dark imagery," wrote Marion in her journal. "The connecting space is the subtle body, the home of the metaphor, the world of soul. That's where I'm working now, visualizing radiant energy transforming into healthy cells. Jung knew psyche and matter were not opposites."

She had a growing awareness that she was somehow trapped—squeezed into too small a space. "I know that this death I am going through has to do with matter that cannot move as quickly as the consciousness that inhabits it. Too much light in too dense matter. My dreams have been telling me that for a year." She had written often about this feeling of being trapped in too small a consciousness.

In our dreams, we are trapped—
In our home,
In a tomb,
In frozen water,
In a sinking ship,
In the stillness,
In the darkness,
In a prison,
In a concentration camp,
In a cave with a rock for a door.

She was trapped in a consciousness that was not yet expansive enough to embrace her new dharma. Where was the block? What, precisely, was split off? What had she not yet gotten big enough to embrace?

Finally, the answer came to her.

What aspect of herself had she exiled? Death.

—— 11 ——

Marion's dharma journey had brought her over and over again to a confrontation with the pairs of opposites: Body and Spirit. Heaven and Hell. Psyche and Soma. Now her dharma—what she liked to call Destiny— would bring her to the final pair of opposites: Life and Death. Could she embrace both life and death at the same time?

This challenge, of course, is precisely the one facing Arjuna at the outset of the Bhagavad Gita. As he quietly surveys the great battlefield of Kurukshetra laid out before him, Arjuna realizes that he is looking squarely at the prospect of his own death. And in the face of this death, he folds. He drops to the floor of his chariot. *I cannot fight this fight.*

It is at this point that Arjuna—terrified—begins "the wondrous dialogue" with Krishna. Krishna begins with a magnificent sermon (and here I paraphrase): "You see Life and Death as opposites," he says to a befuddled Arjuna, "as if you had to choose one over the other. And of course you choose life. But don't you get it? You have to choose both. Life and Death are not enemies. They are not opposites at all. They are inextricably bound to one another. You cannot really choose life without also choosing death."

"Death is inevitable for the living," teaches Krishna. "Birth is inevitable for the dead. Since these are inevitable, you should not sorrow."

All of the Eastern contemplative traditions finally see a full-hearted embrace of death as the very bridge to full life. *Stand at the center and embrace death with your whole heart. Then your work will last forever.*

To our minds this makes no sense. Aren't an embrace of life and an embrace of death mutually exclusive? Krishna teaches that they are not. They are not—not any more than light and dark, mountain and valley, psyche and soma are mutually exclusive. Indeed, holding them both at the same time is what is *required*. It is a sublime paradox.

Paradox is, of course, Marion's home territory. When she looked into the heart of her struggle, Marion discovered her aversion to death. She was trying to keep death out—out of her thoughts, out of her consciousness, out of her dreams. Just as Mom was trying to keep it out. And, alas, as Marion discovered, there is no way to pry loose from the horns of this dilemma but to embrace death fully. Remember that Keats came to exactly the same insight when he finally embraced death as "Life's high meed."

Marion made the decision to embrace death early on in her dance with cancer. She wrote in her journal on January 12, 1994—just months before she came to Kripalu—"I decided if I was going to die, it was all right. Just have to adjust the focus. I realized that Ross and I are living with Death as a daily ally. Death is right here."

—— 12 ——

Marion—along with Jung, along with Krishna—chose a remarkable view of difficulties: Difficulties—even death—are not an enemy from the beyond. They are not an alien force. They are part of the Self. Therefore, what appear to be difficulties are really invitations. They are doorways into a deeper union with split-off parts of the Self. They are opportunities. But in order to make full use of these opportunities, one must be willing to undergo what Marion calls "the initiation."

Marion's awareness that cancer is an *initiation*—not an alien intruder—was a turning point in her journey. In her journal, she pondered the fact that many of the initiations in her life had come precisely through the body. "My body has always been the instrument through which I have been forced to come to consciousness—heatstroke, eating addiction, car accident, kidneys, knees, cancer . . . Its agony forced me onto a new path, where I did not want to go . . . Always through illness God picked me up, dropped me on the new road, and said, 'Walk!'"

Marion saw in her struggle with cancer all the stages of initiation that she had taught for so many years. She describes these stages in *Bone*. Together they make up a stunning reframe of difficulty itself—making it into a path we can fruitfully tread. They include (and here I paraphrase Marion):

- The invitation into the unknown
- The placing of trust in the situation and in one who initiates
- The loss of "the known" and the entry into "the unknown"
- The loss of personal identity
- The fear of the initiation
- Facing the fear
- Active surrender
- The epiphany
- The restoration of personal identity
- The return to the "known world," with more understanding and lived knowledge
- The long integration of the experience into ordinary life

I had heard Marion teach about all of this before, but none of it had come into such focus for me as it did now, reading *Bone*. Initiations are opportunities for us to grow larger. They are death channels. And they are birth channels. They allow us the opportunity to integrate more of our self—more possibility, more reality, more sensation, more feeling. They require everything we've got. They destroy us to re-create us.

These initiations can be terrifying, disorganizing. Writes Marion: "We usually need to leave the old without any promise of the new, need to spend time as forest dwellers, just surviving. Our journey to our old, new home is cyclical, [we must see] that we shall never move in once and for all."

—— 13 ——

Marion teaches that we cannot undergo initiation until we learn to live in paradox. She writes: "We learn to live in paradox, in a world where two apparently exclusive views are held at the same time. In this world, rhythms of paradox are circuitous, slow, born of feeling rising from the thinking heart. Many sense such a place exists. Few talk or walk from it."

Carl Jung created a brilliant developmental strategy for standing in paradox: One must hold both sides of a paradox at the same time, he teaches, without choosing one or the other. Exiling neither. Privileging neither. In this way, we can gradually learn to tolerate living *in the tension of opposites*. Marion states the technique with stunning clarity:

"Holding an inner or outer conflict quietly instead of attempting to resolve it quickly is a difficult idea to entertain. It is even more challenging to experience. However, as Carl Jung believed, if we held the tension between the two opposing forces, there would emerge a third way, which would unite and transcend the two. Indeed, he believed that this transcendent force was crucial to individuation. Whatever the third way is, it usually comes as a surprise, because it has not penetrated our defenses until now. A hasty move to resolve tension can abort growth of the new. If we can hold conflict in psychic utero long enough we can give birth to something new in ourselves."

Hold conflict in psychic utero. This is a skill that can be learned. But it requires a host of collateral skills that most of us in the West have not nurtured: the capacity to stand in mystery; the capacity to tolerate the unknown; the courage to live in the wilderness for a while; the love of the dark and the night and the moon; the wisdom of the circle, not the line. (How can we not hear echoes here of John Keats's Negative Capability?)

Marion teaches that part of our problem is that we try to speed things up—to foreclose them too early; to make them linear; to choose one side over the other. As a result, we do not get the initiation. Not having learned to hold the tension in "psychic utero," we are destined to split the world: Experience becomes either acceptable or unacceptable, good or bad, Life or Death. The initiation fails.

Marion's view allowed her experience with cancer to be full of meaning, to be replete with possibility, and it enabled Death to bring her more deeply into Life. She *got* the initiation.

—— 14 ——

As I think back, I realize that unlike Mom, Dad actually did not go to war with his experience of Alzheimer's. He surrendered gracefully to it. It occurs to me now that somewhere along the way he had learned Marion's lesson. *Stay in the center and embrace death with your whole heart.* Wherever did he learn it? Where had he been initiated into this mystery? Was it fighting on the beaches of Italy during the Second World War? As a kid growing up threadbare in an Ohio River mill town? I remember one night when he cried about his affliction—early on, before the disease was even officially diagnosed. I don't think I had ever seen him cry. His heart was still open. He was able to walk straight ahead, even into Alzheimer's.

Dad surrendered. He opened the door and walked through it. After it was clear that he could no longer live at home, we took him to a very fancy Alzheimer's unit—and then later to a more modest facility nearer to Mom's home. Dad never went to war with this illness. There was some very large capacity in him to face reality.

And I wondered, after his death, if Dad had maybe even thought about the possibility of Alzheimer's—or prepared himself somehow for it. After all, Dad's contracting Alzheimer's should not have been a complete surprise. His mother, my grandmother Cope, had developed the disease, too, in her early sixties—before we even had the name Alzheimer's. I remember my grandmother's suffering all too well. Already deep into the ravages of this disease for which we had no name, she came to live with us for a short while in our little house in Ohio. They are weeks I will never forget. She—my beautiful, sweet grandmother who sang "I'll be Workin' on the Railroad" with us five kids tucked into her big walnut bed in the morning—had become paranoid, confused, disoriented. My family watched, terrified and helpless. One day she chased my mother around the house with a knife—in a fit of paranoid delusion. That very day, she was carted off to Apple Creek State Hospital, where she died—mercifully—just months later, of what the doctors then called "hardening of the arteries."

I remember my father on the afternoon she died—sitting, stunned, at the little telephone stand in the dining room, staring at the blank wall. What had happened to his beautiful, feisty, Scottish mother? She had died in a lunatic asylum. That is what happened, I guess, to Alzheimer's patients before we had the name. On some level, Dad never got over it.

What must it have been like for Dad, then, when he began to experience the same symptoms? What must it have been like for him when he began to forget things? When he could no longer remember how to get from his home to his office? What must it have been like for him, for Dad, who was famous—like his mother—for being always beautifully groomed and turned out? What must it have been like for him when he could no longer figure out how to wear his elegant wardrobe—his Italian shoes, and his English custom suits? When he began to confabulate in order to cover up the fact that he—the historian—no longer knew who was president of the United States?

These questions are very personal for me, as one might imagine. Alzheimer's can be a family disease. My grandmother had it. Then my father. Then my father's only brother. It is probable that one or more of my siblings or I will get it, or some version of it. Will it be me? Maybe it's already lurking there, tangling my innocent brain in knots. Will I be able to adopt Marion's strategy? Should I begin to prepare for it now? Indeed, maybe I *am* preparing for it. Maybe that's what this book is all about. Maybe my concern about living fully—the concern that I laid out at the outset of this book—is driven precisely by this. By death.

— 15 —

Marion survived her initiation through cancer. And I have taught with her many times at Kripalu in the subsequent years. She wrote at the end of *Bone* that she had "died into life." And I believe it. Our workshops together are so much fun. They are full of dancing and singing. They have included poetry readings with Robert Bly—digging deep into the dream world of participants and dancing with them to the music of Frédéric Chopin and Richard Strauss. Marion does it up grand: She usually emerges on the Saturday evenings of our workshops in a long gold lamé dress, and reads Emily Dickinson and John Keats and Shakespeare to the hundreds of participants. In our individual work during these workshops, Marion has participants digging around in the muck and the earth of their inner worlds. I have been transformed by the process of working with her. And my relationship to the dream world has never been the same.

Marion looks older now. Months of radiation therapy have left damage throughout her body. One winter after leaving Kripalu she fell on the way home and fractured both legs—bones already weakened by therapy for cancer. She endured months of rehabilitation. Yet when she next appeared at Kripalu to teach with me, she was still dancing.

"An aged man is but a paltry thing," wrote William Butler Yeats, one of Marion's favorite poets.

An aged man is but a paltry thing,
A wretched coat upon a stick, unless
Soul clap its hands and sing, and louder sing
For every tatter in its mortal dress,

Unless Soul clap its hands and sing! There is a way to live beyond the pairs of opposites—beyond gain and loss, hope and fear, praise and blame, fame and ill-repute. And the Soul already knows the way. We must follow. The sage who lives like this, says Krishna—the sage who lives beyond the pairs of opposites—"awakens to the light in the night of all creatures."

Initiation by cancer became for Marion a new birth canal. "Cancer has made me sadder and wiser," she wrote, "and therefore richer. Because death is an essential part of life, to be fully alive is to be prepared for it. The gift of cancer is the gift of NOW. . . . Through failures, symptoms, problems, we are prodded to renounce attachments, redundant now. With the breakdown of what has gone before, the possibility of rebirth comes."

— 16 —

Toward the end of her initiation through cancer, Marion and Ross were at a friend's fiftieth birthday party. Everyone was dancing. Marion was glued to the couch. Doctor's orders: fragile bones! Finally, she said to Ross, "Come on, Ross, let's dance."

"Oh, Marion," he says, "you know you can't dance. You could break your back."

"I sit out the polka," she writes in her journal, describing the exasperating moment, "can't keep my feet still."

"A voice comes up from my perineum," she writes with increasing fervor, " 'Marion, you can sit on this couch until you rot, but I am going to dance. I don't care what Ross thinks . . . I don't care what anybody thinks. I don't care if you break your back. I don't care if you drop down dead. I am going to dance! I am going to live!' I feel the archetypal energy lifting me off the couch, propelling me across the room—I feel it pushing through my benumbed feet, legs, thighs, torso, arms, hands, through every cell into my head. It is TOTAL. I feel myself Gypsy—a twenty-four-year-old glowing woman. I am being danced. People are gazing at me aghast, probably thinking, 'This old lady sat on the couch all evening; suddenly she's transformed into a hands-in-the-air Gypsy. What's she up to?' Do I care?

"Then a stranger—a Dutchman who has just arrived—catches my vision, jumps into my circle, and we dance a dance as fierce as I have ever danced before. If my back breaks, if I drop dead, it doesn't matter. I am twenty-four. I am healthy. I am whole."

TEN

Ludwig van Beethoven:
Turn the Wound into Light

My piano teacher, Douglas, noticed it right away: "You seem to have a special relationship with that piece of music," he mused one evening during my weekly lesson.

Douglas was referring to one of Ludwig van Beethoven's masterful final three piano sonatas—the Sonata in A-flat, op. 110—which I was manifestly butchering in front of him at our lesson every Tuesday night. Who knows why he had given me this complex piece to study? I wasn't technically ready for it. (Douglas told me later that he "just had a hunch.") But I fell in love with this sonata almost immediately, and I soon determined—perversely, I guess—to master it. I never did.

The first movement was easy going. The sonata starts with a tender theme and variations in A-flat—calm and bright, like a sunny day on a sparkling pond. Things soon get darker, however. After the sweetest of introductions comes an "Arioso Dolente"—a sorrowful song. It is inexpressibly sad. This song is followed by a complex fugue in which Beethoven seems to be struggling to come to terms with his sorrow—to master it. The fugue is wild, long, and fierce, and learning it just about drove me out of my mind. Beethoven works back and forth between the beautiful song and the groaning fugal structure, all the while becoming more and more impassioned. The theme of the fugue works against itself, at times coming a hairsbreadth from flying apart. There is no question: Beethoven is bringing everything he has to this effort. This is a life-and-death struggle of some kind. The fugue, insanely complex at its zenith, finally finds an ecstatic and harmonious conclusion. The performer collapses, exhausted.

OK, I thought. This was crazy, wonderful stuff. I could feel Beethoven working away at something here—turning the theme upside down and inside out, breaking it apart in strange ways—fracturing it. This music was really getting under my skin, and I could feel my resolve to master it rise. I practiced this sonata intensively for months. I broke it down measure by measure; I studied its structure; I spent hours working out my own ham-handed fingerings for complex passages; I played it over and over again to Douglas's withering critique.

The more I got to know this piece, the more passionate I became about it, and the more I fell in love with Beethoven. Any time I dipped into this sonata, I felt Beethoven's presence. There he was. When I was a kid, I had learned to play the piano by placing my small hands on top of my grandfather's as he played his beautiful ballads. Now my hands were on Beethoven's. Through Beethoven's music, I *knew* him—in the Keatsean sense. This was not just music. It was transmission.

Douglas's hunch had been right: There was something important for me in this music. It took me on a journey into some untamed part of myself. It reminded me a little of Thoreau's description of his discovery of "the Wild" after he climbed Mount Katahdin in Maine. This contact with "the Wild" changed Thoreau and his view of nature forever. He discovered nature to be rough, untamed, dangerous, relentlessly itself, and shockingly disdainful of human laws. Thoreau declared that human beings could not be fully human without "the Wild." Beethoven, it seemed, was a Mount Katahdin experience for me.

As a young poet, Emily Dickinson wrote to her soon-to-be mentor, Thomas Wentworth Higginson, and sent him several poems to examine. At the end of the letter, she queried: "Are you too deeply occupied to say if my Verse is alive?" Higginson was thunderstruck by her poems. "Your poetry lives!" he wrote back immediately. "It lives." Just so with Beethoven's music. It lives. W*ork performed in the thrall of dharma has a life of its own.* It has an existence strangely independent of its author.

— 2 —

Ludwig van Beethoven is the apotheosis of the dharma project. *If you bring forth what is within you it will save you.* If any man was ever saved by his dharma, it was surely Beethoven.

Beethoven was an emotionally wounded, profoundly neurotic man, who was tortured by inner conflicts throughout his life. He suffered from the very kinds of internal divisions that Marion had described— split between his massive idealism about human nature on the one hand and the misanthropic, angry, spiteful man that he could be on the other. He was split between the ecstatic and spiritualized writer of the *Missa Solemnis* and the solitary man who wandered the streets of Vienna at night in search of prostitutes. And as with most neurotics, he was tortured by his own behavior. Beethoven was suicidal off and on for significant periods of time throughout his life. And even in his most stable periods, he could appear to be just on the brink of madness.

Yet, split as he had been throughout life, as Beethoven lay on his deathbed he was a fulfilled man. Not a happy man, mind you. But a fulfilled man—certainly. (There can be a world of difference between happiness and fulfillment. Even as he lay dying, Beethoven purportedly raised a fist to heaven.) Beethoven was a man who had found his dharma, and had brought everything he had to it. "I have run the race," said St. Paul toward the end of his long career as an Apostle. "I have kept the faith." Beethoven might have made the same declaration.

This fragile, driven, and tenderhearted man was, in the final analysis, a saved man. He had been saved by his work. In the midst of an almost unbearably painful life, God dropped Beethoven a lifeline: music. And Beethoven reached for it with everything he had.

Beethoven was in love with his dharma. Unhappy as he was in life, he felt an urgent calling to fully express the gift that was in him. It was a reason to live. He several times wrote, in effect, I would have killed myself, but I had work to do. "Before my departure for the Elysian fields," Beethoven wrote to a friend, midway through his life, "I must leave behind me what the Eternal Spirit has infused into my soul and bids me complete . . ."

And now a surprise: Beethoven was deeply inspired by his reading of the Bhagavad Gita.

(When I discovered this I almost fell off my chair. Beethoven knew about yoga? My worlds had collided. This discovery caused me to call a dharma buddy in Paris out of the blue—and practically in the middle of the night—to tell him this news.)

In his search for psychological and spiritual survival, Beethoven had combed the world's great literature. And perhaps not surprisingly, he had bumped into the Bhagavad Gita. He read it intensively. He made notes from it—and from other great Hindu scriptures—and kept these sacred phrases in plain view under glass on his desk.

By the age of twenty-eight, Beethoven had discovered the idea of a holy dharma—a holy work that would save him. He realized that it was imperative that his life be spent manifesting his gift. He scribbled the following quote from the Bhagavad Gita into his personal diary: "Blessed is the man who, having subdued all his passions, performeth with his active faculties all the functions of life, unconcerned about the event . . . Be not one whose motive for action is the hope of reward. Perform thy duty, abandon all thought of the consequence, and make the event equal, whether it terminate in good or evil; for such an equality is called yoga." And, as we will see, in his quest to make meaning of his suffering, Beethoven enacted in his life virtually all the pillars of Krishna's teaching.

Most interesting to me in Beethoven's particularly vivid dharma story is the way in which *authentic dharma turns suffering into light.* Dharma did not end Beethoven's suffering. He suffered until the end of his life. I have at home a picture of him on his deathbed, a man utterly worn out by his suffering. But through his dharma, Beethoven transformed his suffering. By the middle of his life, he had learned to plumb the depths of his agony, and to use it. He had learned to open his many wounds—his deafness, his craziness, his paranoid suspicions—to the full view of humanity, and to let a strange light pour from them.

Beethoven would abhor even the slightest hint of comparison to Christ—Beethoven, who seemed so very un-Christlike, and who eschewed much of Catholic doctrine and dogma. But in fact he was the very image of "the suffering servant" described by St. Paul in the New

Testament. When I think of Beethoven as I have come to understand him, I cannot but see in my mind's eye those vivid Catholic images of Christ with his palms and side oozing blood and light. Both blood *and* light, mind you. Beethoven's relentless—and often bloody—pursuit of his dharma gave light to the world. It saved him. But it also saved the world. More about this strange fact later.

Ultimately, as Beethoven's great biographer, Maynard Solomon, has written, "Beethoven turned all of his defeats into victories." This would be a good thing for each of us to learn. We each have wounds. Can a full performance of our dharma turn our wounds into light?

— 3 —

The few verifiable accounts of Beethoven's childhood are devastating to read. Beethoven's father, Johann, was a mediocre, insecure, and alcoholic court musician, who bullied his son (young "Louis," as he was called) into musical training when he was only four or five years old. Johann's instruction of Louis was brutal, willful, abusive, and demeaning. One family friend routinely "saw the little Louis van Beethoven in the house standing in front of the clavier and weeping."

As a child, Beethoven was used in the most cynical way. His father apparently viewed the boy's talents as a significant source of income and also as a potential means of reflected glory. To make matters worse, there is no record that his mother, Maria Magdalena, defended her son from this ongoing abuse. Indeed, the accounts indicate that she was herself neglectful: "[The] Beethoven children were not delicately brought up," recounts one witness. "They were often left with maids . . . and Beethoven himself was often dirty and [neglected]."

What is perhaps most perverse is that Beethoven's father attempted to willfully quash young Beethoven's tremendous early inventiveness and creativity at the piano. From a very early age, Beethoven was brilliantly adept at improvisation—on both the clavier and the violin. This kind of improvisation was the hallmark of the great nineteenth century virtuosos and composers, so one would have thought a father who hoped to cash in would have helped to promote this incipient genius. Not, alas, the hapless, cruel, and bungling Johann.

Interestingly, the adult Beethoven was absolutely mute on the subject of his early years. But it is clear that by our contemporary standards young Louis had suffered an abusive childhood, and could be expected to suffer lifelong symptoms of what we would today call post-traumatic stress disorder. Indeed, that is exactly what happened: Young Beethoven became shy and reclusive; he was often monosyllabic; he was socially inept and maladroit; he had difficulty maintaining basic standards of self-care and cleanliness.

But Beethoven had one thin lifeline to sanity and personal restitution: his music. However cruelly it was initially administered to him, music nonetheless came to provide him with a protected inner world into which he could retreat. His happiest hours were when the family was away, and he was free to practice and improvise at the clavier. From an early age he engaged in intensive practice, which was a kind of play that helped him reconstitute himself. Indeed, it was the only form of play open to him, and he gobbled it up hungrily.

Intensive practice provided Beethoven with the tools to symbolically and energetically transform his experience. It gave him an increasing experience of self-efficacy and self-esteem, and provided him with an experience of *fun*. Finally, it came to provide him with a profound sense of purpose, accomplishment, and meaning. It turns out that these qualities of dharma can rescue even a life in peril.

Later in his life, Beethoven (on rare occasions) shared memories of his early days with his student Carl Czerny. He described how he had practiced prodigiously—even at five, six, seven years old—usually until well past midnight. We can see now that Beethoven had begun at a very tender age to enter into the phase of mastery we have called "deliberate practice." His early efforts had all of the hallmarks: He practiced in chunks of four hours; he practiced *with the intention of improving his performance*; he broke complex musical tasks down into their component parts; whenever he could, he used trainers and teachers—and all kinds of feedback—to improve. Young Beethoven hungered for instruction, and sought it out wherever he could find it.

Beethoven's early practice was more than play. It was, indeed, as Robert Frost has written, "play for mortal stakes." It allowed him to find his center—an inner bulwark that he would use to survive adulthood.

— 4 —

Young Louis was a bizarre, awkward kid. Strangely, for a musical prod-igy, he was what we might call a klutz, both emotionally and physically. He was forever knocking things over, breaking things, inadvertently de-stroying things. He could, by all accounts, be hugely irritating to be around. But many saw underneath his awkward exterior a sweetness and tenderness.

The boy had suffered. And so he was understandably touched by the sufferings of others. Throughout life, he identified with the misery of friends and acquaintances, and he felt called to help when he could. He saw his music as the best kind of help he could offer. In a letter of 1811, he writes: "From my earliest childhood my zeal to serve our poor suffer-ing humanity in any way whatsoever by means of my art has made no compromise with any lower motive." And he later wrote, "Since I was a child my greatest happiness and pleasure have been to be able to do something for others."

In addition to music, the gods sent young Beethoven another saving gift: a noble, trustworthy, and kind mentor. Christian Gottlob Neefe was Beethoven's first real teacher, and he helped rescue him in many of the same ways that Charles Cowden Clarke rescued the young John Keats. Neefe was a good musician. But more important for Beethoven, he was a good man. Beethoven was starved for the kind of positive regard Neefe offered. For the first time in his life, Beethoven was *seen*. His talent, his genius, his strong determination, his resilience—these qualities were seen, appreciated, and reflected to him.

In his late teens, and probably as a result of Neefe's coaching, Beethoven began to read widely and voraciously. This is when he began to frame his life as *a quest to understand*. He read poetry, drama, phi-losophy of all kinds. "There is hardly any treatise which could be too learned for me," he declared.

Beethoven was not an intellectual. His quest was more urgent than that. He was grasping for psychological survival. "I have not the slightest pretension to what is properly called erudition. Yet from my childhood I have striven to understand *what the better and wiser people* of every age were driving at in their works." This was not a pose. Beethoven was never interested in high-blown metaphysics, but only in practical solutions to the problems of living. This quality of inquiry marks him as a real yogi. He might have said, as Thoreau did, "even I am at times a yogi."

— 5 —

As we have seen, Beethoven had begun his phase of deliberate practice by the time he was five or six. By the time he was fifteen he was a brilliant and virtuosic pianist. And by his late teens he was probably the greatest pianist in Europe—the successor to Mozart, who had been dead just twelve months when Beethoven arrived in Vienna. Beethoven was highly sought after in the palaces and salons of aristocratic connoisseurs. Some were offended by the sheer boldness and unconventionality of his musical style, but most describe his musical presence as positively astonishing. We have this eyewitness account written by Carl Czerny:

> "In whatever company he might chance to be, he knew how to produce such an effect upon every hearer that frequently not an eye remained dry, while many would break out into loud sobs; for there was something wonderful in his expression in addition to the beauty and originality of his ideas and his spirited style of rendering them."

No doubt about it: Beethoven was a wunderkind. And he knew it. He aimed to be the best. He took on all comers. He frequently participated in pianistic duels, in which he challenged other important European pianists of his day to public competitions. These were like great athletic competitions and they sometimes drew hundreds of spectators. Beethoven always won. (One sore loser, Abbé Joseph Gelinek, believed that Beethoven's supernormal powers at the piano could only be explained as sorcery—and the good Abbé later described being "bested by that young fellow [Beethoven] who must be in league with the devil.")

Beethoven was by all accounts a commanding presence, though often in a positively unnerving fashion. Solomon gives us a description: "[He] was short of stature, with a large head, and thick black hair that framed a pock-marked face. His forehead was broad and heavily underlined by bushy eyebrows." Many found him ugly. But everyone noticed the unusual beauty and expressiveness of his eyes, which were sometimes flashing with life, other times inexpressively sad. Solomon continues: "His mouth was small and delicately shaped. He had white teeth, which he habitually rubbed with a napkin or handkerchief . . . He was powerfully built, with wide shoulders, strong hands overgrown with hair, and short, thick fingers."

There was a crudeness in Beethoven's appearance that all witnesses remark upon. He could be unpolished even when decked out in finery. But his friends found him often exuberant, lively, and talkative. Czerny remembered him as "always merry, mischievous, full of witticisms and jokes." Nonetheless, all contemporary accounts also remark on his moodiness, his emotional fragility, and a tendency toward melancholy.

Beethoven clung heroically to his life's work. There is absolutely no question that he understood that music would be his only path to wholeness. He understood the meaning of his gift. And he felt a profound responsibility to it. He knew that he could not live as other people lived. "Live only in your art," he wrote in his diary, "for you are so limited by your senses. This is nevertheless the *only existence* for you."

Beethoven understood that if he were to survive, he would have to privilege his art—his dharma—above all other activities in life. He would, in fact, have to pare away everything that was *not* his art. This evidenced a solid understanding of Krishna's doctrine of unity of purpose. "Everything that is called life should be sacrificed to the sublime and be a sanctuary of art," Beethoven wrote in his diary.

As a result of this view, Beethoven created a life that was organized in every way to support his dharma. His daily schedule is instructive. He rose at daybreak, ate breakfast, and went directly to his desk, where he worked until midday. After lunch he ordinarily took a long walk—sometimes twice around the city—which could occupy a good part of the afternoon. This walking practice is redolent of Thoreau, of Frost, and indeed of many great writers. Beethoven discovered that his most productive work hours were in the morning, and so he protected this time, and made sure that he arrived fresh at his desk in the morning, ready to commune with his muse. He usually retired to bed early.

Beethoven pared away what most of us think of as "fun," but the truth of the matter is that there was nothing more fun for him than his music. He sketched musical ideas constantly, whether at home, on the street, in a tavern, or lying on his side in a meadow. "I always have a notebook . . . with me, and when an idea comes to me, I put it down at once," he told young Gerhard von Breuning. "I even get up in the middle of the night when a thought comes, because otherwise I might forget it." He filled a vast number of notebooks during his lifetime, and retained them for reference until his death.

—— 6 ——

Work was a kind of sustaining play for Beethoven. But what exactly was he working on? Nothing small or insignificant. He was attempting nothing less than mastery of the entire Western musical tradition.

By the time he was in his midtwenties, Beethoven had mastered the tools and vernacular of the greatest living musical masters: Haydn (his teacher for a time) and Mozart. Early in his career, Beethoven had taken on an intensive study of the forms and patterns of the Western classical tradition. He had, in particular, begun a close study of the central form of this tradition—what we today call sonata form.

Sonata form was the organizing paradigm of Western music. This form, carefully developed over the course of centuries, helped a composer develop the logic of a piece of music. Sonata form was organized around three main components: the exposition of a theme, or the declaration of a musical "argument" embedded in a harmonic structure; the gradual development of some of the interesting possibilities inherent in that harmonic structure and direction; and, finally, the recapitulation of the theme and harmonic structure—now transformed and deepened in some important way. This form provided a brilliant way of developing a musical thought—investigating its possibilities and bringing it to a resolution or conclusion. Most important, it created a container for all the components of drama: for creating and sustaining tension, for expressing development and transformation, for giving us the feeling of forward movement. Sonata form is a remarkably psychological approach to music. It connects us with something quintessentially human.

Sigmund Freud himself would have appreciated the possibilities for "working through" psychological conflict that are inherent in sonata form. Freud, of course, called this conflict "neurosis." Neurosis is simply *conflict between parts of the self*—conflict, say, between our desires and our conscience; or conflict between our sometimes monstrously driven cravings and our more prudent selves, or even conflict between an overweening scrupulosity and normal human wishes.

All of the most mature forms of human play involve us in the "working through" of these conflicts. When "work is play for mortal stakes," as it was for Beethoven, it helps us to resolve doubt and division, and to at least briefly experience a sense of resolution, of "union," and of wellbeing.

So, sonata form provided Beethoven with an effective form for working through his inner conflicts. Some might protest that this working through was only symbolic. It was in fact very, very real. The working through provided to Beethoven by his music was central to his psychological survival. It was essential that Beethoven plumb the depths of musical form, because in doing so he was plumbing his own depths.

Piano sonatas were Beethoven's first laboratory for investigating the transformational possibilities of sonata form. Through his development of the piano sonata, he was able to investigate the plasticity of sonata form itself. What was the form's real capacity for holding conflict? For helping him endure the tension of opposites? How much of himself could he pour into this form?

We have said that deliberate practice leads to heightened pattern recognition. There is no greater example of this heightened pattern recognition than Beethoven, who found astonishing new patterns within the structure of Western music. He found patterns within patterns, just as Thoreau did in nature and Corot did in painting. Beethoven found within the sonata form new, unexplored possibilities. As Solomon tells us, he explored "thematic condensation; more intense, extended and dramatic development; and the infusion of richer fantasy and improvisatory materials into an even more highly structured classicism." Beethoven saw possibilities in this form that only a highly developed musical imagination could perceive.

In effect, then, Beethoven became a musical seer. Like the mystical *rishis* of ancient India, he perceived aspects of reality that were beyond the perceptual range of ordinary people. Very few of his contemporaries could understand the musical leaps he had made. And of course, not seeing the genius of his refined perception, his critics called him "mad."

They were only half right. Throughout his life, Beethoven was indeed constantly threatened by the forces of disintegration planted in his childhood. But his music became a laboratory in which he could bring these forces to the surface, work them out, master them. This is the very hallmark of great dharma. Each of us must find the form that allows this naming, this working through, and, finally, this mastery. We may find these forms in sports, in the arts, in finance, in academia, in relationship building, in child-rearing—or, indeed, in stamp collecting. *But find them we must.*

— 7 —

By his midtwenties, at the very apex of his meteoric rise to the top of musical Vienna, Beethoven was harboring a devastating secret. He was slowly going deaf. He had no idea what this might mean for his music. It was clear that he would no longer be able to conduct or perform. But would he even be able to compose? Beethoven was justly afraid that he might not be able to psychologically survive the loss of his creative life. In an effort to deny his increasing infirmity—both to others and to himself—he became more and more withdrawn. His social and emotional isolation added an almost unbearable burden to an already heavily stressed psyche. His fragile compromise with life was breaking down.

Beethoven describes his increasing misery in a now-famous letter to his friend Franz Wegeler: ". . . my ears continue to hum and buzz day and night. I must confess that I lead a miserable life. For almost two years I have ceased to attend any social functions, just because I find it impossible to say to people: I am deaf. If I had any other profession I might be able to cope with my infirmity; but in my profession it is a terrible handicap . . . Heaven only knows what is to become of me. Already I have often cursed my Creator and my existence."

Ludwig van Beethoven had made a fragile compromise with life. Now the whole house of cards was threatening to collapse. As his deafness increased, so did his anxiety, his dread, and his depression.

In the spring of 1802, Beethoven moved to the quiet little village of Heiligenstadt, north of Vienna on the Danube, where he apparently remained for almost half a year. This move had been suggested by a physician, who assured him that a period of enforced rest and quiet would make a difference in his hearing. When it became clear that even radical quiet was not having the slightest positive effect, he began to unravel. In Heiligenstadt—alone, desperate, despairing—he seriously contemplated suicide. He most likely remained at serious risk of taking his own life for a period of some weeks, or even months.

Throughout the course of this ordeal, the composer searched his own soul. He raged at heaven. He prayed. He most likely wrote in his journal—though we have no writing from the very center of this crisis. What we do have, miraculously, is a document that Beethoven wrote after he had finally made the decision to live. It is a remarkable piece of personal testimony—now known as the Heiligenstadt Testament—in which he bares his soul to his family and his friends. The Testament, written in the form of a letter to his brothers, was never mailed. It was discovered in his desk drawer after his death.

The Heiligenstadt Testament recounts Beethoven's wrestling match with suicidality. It describes the razor's edge on which he then lived, and makes a full accounting of the consequences—both personal and professional—of his deafness. And it describes his decision to go on living. He would live, henceforth, he says, *for his art alone:* "It was only my art that held me back [from suicide] . . . Ah, it seemed to me impossible to leave the world until I had brought forth all that I felt was within me. So I endured this wretched existence . . . Patience, they say, is what I must now choose for my guide, and I have done so—Perhaps I shall get better, perhaps not; I am ready.—Forced to become a philosopher already in my twenty-eighth year.—Divine One, thou seest my inmost soul; thou knowest that therein dwells the love of mankind and the desire to do good . . ."

Beethoven had faced death. And he had decided to live. As a result of this ordeal, he was less afraid of either death or suffering. The experience of utter despair profoundly changed him. "Stay in the center and embrace death with your whole heart," says the *Tao te Ching*, as you will recall. Though Beethoven had not discovered the *Tao te Ching* in his vast reading of Eastern literature, nevertheless, he had independently discovered this same principle of dharma. *Embrace death with your whole heart and you will endure forever*

"With joy I hasten to meet death," he writes toward the end of the Heiligenstadt Testament. "—If it comes before I have had the chance to develop all my artistic capacities, it will still be coming too soon despite my harsh fate, and I should probably wish it later—yet even so I should be happy, for would it not free me from a state of endless suffering?"

Beethoven finished his Testament with a strange good-bye, "Thus I bid thee farewell," he ends. To whom was he saying good-bye? It seems clear that he was saying good-bye to an *earlier version of himself.*

In the years leading up to Heiligenstadt, Beethoven had angrily railed against the injustice of his condition. He was Job with his fist raised toward Heaven. But for the most part during those earlier years, he kept his despair a secret. He confided it to no one. He intended to use his anger to keep him alive, to keep his creative spirit moving. He would overcome. "I will take Fate by the throat," he had declared.

Now, at Heiligenstadt, came a great surrender. And not just a surrender to a terrible fate, but a true acceptance of that fate. At first, of course, his surrender looked more like resignation. But at Heiligenstadt, he found the beginnings of a true acceptance of his situation. After Heiligenstadt there was a deep change in Beethoven. He had discovered the link between his suffering and his art. His sacrifice now had meaning. He had discovered one of the central principles of dharma.

By the end of the summer of 1802, as J. W. N. Sullivan tells us, Beethoven had discovered that his work was mightier than his suffering. He had discovered, in fact, that his work could not be destroyed by his suffering: ". . . he found that his genius, that he had felt called upon to cherish and protect, was really a mighty force using him as a channel or servant . . . only when the consciously defiant Beethoven had succumbed, only when his pride and strength had been so reduced that he was willing, even eager, to die and abandon the struggle, did he find that his creative power was indeed indestructible and that it was its deathless energy that made it impossible for him to die."

"In the middle of winter I at last discovered that there was in me an invincible summer," wrote Albert Camus, in the midst of a similar period of despair. *An invincible summer.*

"Never again was [Beethoven's] attitude toward life one of defiance," writes Sullivan. "He had become aware within himself of an indomitable creative energy that nothing could destroy." Beethoven, exulting in this newfound freedom, wrote the following note to himself in the margins of his great C Major string quartet, "In the same way that you are now able to throw yourself into the whirlpool of society, so you are able to write your works in spite of all social hindrances. Let your deafness no longer be a secret—even for art."

Beethoven came to see that complete surrender to his situation in life—to his deafness, to his various neuroses—was absolutely essential for his own spiritual development and for the development of his art. He accepted the apparent mystery that his art and his suffering were inextricably linked.

— 8 —

After Heiligenstadt, Beethoven's creativity burst forth, unrestrained, at least temporarily, by inner conflict. Having worked through a nearly fatal series of doubts and self-division, Beethoven entered a period of unity of purpose and of certitude. "I live entirely in my music," he wrote, "and hardly have I completed one composition when I have already begun another. At my present rate of composition, I often produce three or four works at the same time." This burgeoning of creativity reminds us of Thoreau at Walden, of Frost in England, or of Whitman after the Civil War. The music, Beethoven says, seems to be writing itself. The Master now experienced a new dimension of trust in The Gift. He understood that his gift was not personal. That he was not the Doer. That his responsibility was not to *create* The Gift—that was a done deal—but only to sustain it, to husband it, to nurture it in every way possible. This newfound faith in The Gift had a paradoxical effect: It *relaxed* him and *energized* him at one and the same time.

What emerged next was what some biographers call Beethoven's "heroic period." The term "heroic" is usually thought to refer to Beethoven's fascination with power, and with powerful men—specifically Napoleon, to whom he had first dedicated his magisterial Third Symphony, the *Eroica*. In fact, "heroic" refers to Beethoven's own newly exuberant experience of faith.

Beethoven now truly began to intuit the connection between The Wound and The Gift. He would never again try to cover up The Wound. In fact, he would open it for all to see. He would submit to the mystery of his fate, and trust it. He would allow himself to be a sacrifice. "Submission, deepest submission to your fate, only this can give you the sacrifices—for this matter of service," he wrote in his *Tagebuch* (his diary). What does this mean? The theme of sacrifice and submission colors many of his entries in the *Tagebuch* henceforward. It means that he accepts his life as a sacrifice. But now a *willing sacrifice*. Even an eager one. He began to understand that The Wound itself is an aspect of The Gift. They cannot be divided.

Solomon grasps this essential point: "Like Henry James's obscure hurt and Dostoevsky's holy disease, even [Beethoven's] loss of hearing was in some sense necessary or at least useful, to the fulfillment of his creative quest." Mysteriously, The Gift issues forth out of The Wound. It does not quite heal The Wound, *but it makes sense of it.* It gives it meaning. And meaning is everything.

With this newfound understanding, Beethoven now perceived altogether new possibilities in sonata form—precisely for giving voice to The Wound. Sonata form had not yet been stretched to its capacity—to express either heroic or tragic levels of experience. But Beethoven now saw that it was uniquely suited to this task. He grasped (as Solomon tells us) "its unique ability simultaneously to release and to contain the most explosive musical concepts within binding aesthetic structures."

Krishna and Arjuna give us the field of battle. Is this just a symbol? No, it is not. It is quite real. The battlefield is an absolutely central component of the Gita. Our conflicts and inner divisions—all that separates us from our true selves—must be worked out on the field of real life. On the field of relationships. Of work. Of effort. Of hobbies. Of callings. This is what dharma is. Dharma calls us not to just any old battlefield, but to the battlefield where we will suffer most fruitfully. Where our suffering will be most useful to ourselves, to our souls, and to the world.

The ongoing argument in Bhagavad Gita scholarship about whether the battlefield at Kurukshetra is symbolic or real is a red herring. The battlefield is both entirely *symbolic* and entirely *real.* This is the genius of Krishna's teaching on action. The soul must be purified through action. Beethoven gives us another kind of field of battle, in which great forces fight with one another, and in which dharma, truth, and unity eventually triumph.

Beethoven's battleground is harmony and theme and variations. Music itself becomes a way of working through soul-shattering conflict. His own desperate need to work through his inner divisions gave the world a wholly new way of working with the problem of doubt and despair.

—— 9 ——

Beethoven's fragile compromise with life broke down one more time before his death. Between the years 1815 and 1820, he survived a series of devastating psychological challenges: the severe illness of his brother Caspar Carl; the threatened loss of his nephew—and "adoptive son"— Karl (and with it the loss of his fantasy of "family"); the loss of his dream of marriage and the final renunciation of his hopes for domestic happiness.

Once again, Beethoven was on the brink of despair, and he found himself on the edge of emotional breakdown. His suicidal impulses were reawakened, and he talked of suicide with his friends and companions. "I often despair and would like to die," he wrote. During this period, his physical appearance once again deteriorated, and his friends took to buying him new clothes—trying in vain to clean him up. On one now-famous occasion he was almost arrested in Vienna as a vagrant. "I learned yesterday," wrote a Viennese acquaintance, "that Beethoven had become crazy."

During these years, Beethoven was again at times close to the breaking point. Many of his symptoms were precisely what we might expect of a man who had been profoundly traumatized as a boy, and who had had no help to integrate this trauma: He had sudden rages, experienced increasing obsessive states (especially around money), felt unreasonably persecuted, and experienced ungrounded suspicions. He was in some ways—as Vienna saw daily—"a sublime madman."

And yet, underneath these outward signs and symptoms was still percolating the very best of Beethoven—his capacity to use his work to survive, and to transmute his suffering into sublime creations.

During these years, Beethoven embarked on a new phase of his spiritual journey. He read voraciously, studying the core scriptures of many of the world's great religions. He discussed his existential questions with a small circle of friends, through the vehicle of his "Conversation Books." He developed a series of notebooks through which he communicated with his friends—intimates who were some of Vienna's leading citizens, writers, philosophers, musicians, civil servants, journalists. He investigated various views of God. Above all, during these difficult years, Beethoven increased his sense of dedication to his own duty. "God sees into my innermost heart and knows that as a man I perform most conscientiously and on all occasions the duties which Humanity, God and Nature enjoin upon me . . ." Humanity, God, and Nature: These became Beethoven's spiritual pillars.

What rose in Beethoven now was an intense determination to bring forth the best that was within him. He set to work. He knew that he would not have time to finish all of the fantastic musical creations that he had already envisioned. He knew that he was in a race against time. But he was determined to bring forth what he could. "I must leave behind me what the Eternal Spirit has infused into my soul," he wrote. "Why, I feel as if I had hardly composed more than a few notes."

Beethoven identified with Arjuna's doubt and questioning, and with the idea of action that is redemptive. He copied into his diary a number of Krishna's teachings about dharma: "Perform thy duty! Abandon all thought of the consequence." Beethoven had understood Krishna's lesson: Your soul can be saved only through *action in the performance of your own dharma*. He had copied another pillar of Krishna's teachings into his diary: "Let not thy life be spent in inaction! Depend upon application!" And so, the Master launched into his final period of action. What emerged was another astonishing period of productivity.

Beethoven was remarkably clearheaded in mapping out the work that he wished to finish before his death: There was the great Ninth Symphony, of course; the *Missa Solemnis;* his spectacularly modern *Diabelli Variations;* and of course his late string quartets. He put his work above everything and organized his life exclusively around it. "My motto is always: *nulla dies sine linea* [no day without a line] . . . and if I let my Muse go to sleep, it is only that she may be all the more active when she awakes. I still hope to create a few great works, and then like an old child to finish my earthly course somewhere among kind people . . ."

In his search to fully express the sublime music he now heard in his head, Beethoven scoured the history of Western music. He turned backward in his final years toward Bach and Handel, toward the earlier geniuses of fugue and polyphony. What resulted was a remarkable final maturation of his style. In his last several years, we see Beethoven making new connections—expanding sonata form to its very breaking point. His creations were thrilling to those few who could understand what he was doing. And for those who could *not* understand it, he had little use.

Beethoven was now fiercely determined to offer his final contribution to mankind. He dedicated himself wholly to work. He stripped his life down to absolute essentials. He let go of social niceties. He cared not what others thought. He withdrew into himself when necessary. (And he found a rationale for this turn inward—yogis call this "introversion"— in the literature of the world's great religions. As he himself wrote in his journals, he discovered the kind of deep meditative states and ritual silence described by Brahmin novices. Time both slowed down and speeded up. He became, indeed, a yogi, during these last years— experiencing a decided maturation of his mind, of his capacity to focus, and of his capacity to perceive subtle patterns in musical forms, patterns that few of his contemporaries could perceive or understand.

It was, indeed, Beethoven's late-in-life genius that I had experienced in my struggle with his piano sonata opus 110. In this sonata, Beethoven was working through The Wound with such fierceness and with such skill that his arresting musical design caught me up in its net. There was something new and dangerous here that reached far down into my soul to touch my own Gordian knots—and my own longing for freedom. It was indeed the music of a Seer: wildly free, though brilliantly married with form.

Beethoven's music has changed my life. What has it given me? It has given me not only inspiration and hope, but a visceral way to work through my own neurotic conflicts—a path through my own inner tangles. Every time I play his sonata, I touch a part of myself that nothing else can reach. And afterward, I have the distinct feeling of having been sorted out. Beethoven, in working through his own suffering with integrity, has carried some kind of load for me. This is the mystical effect of dharma.

It is this very effect that we see shining forth from the lives we have examined in this book so far. It shines forth from Marion. From Keats. From Thoreau. From Anthony. Each one of them was able to discover the secret of turning his own particular wound into light—and a light that illumined not only their own lives, but the life of the world.

—— 10 ——

Toward the close of his life, a fantastic transformation took place in Beethoven. The more Beethoven became vulnerable to the deterioration of age—both psychologically and physically—the more his Soul clapped its hands . . . and louder sang.

Two remarkable sketches survive of Beethoven on his deathbed—one by Joseph Teltscher drawn rapidly just before Beethoven's death, and another by Josef Danhauser drawn just after his death. Both portray a man who is entirely spent. Spent, yes. But like Hokusai on his deathbed, still wanting to get up and work.

Solomon describes the moment of his death: "Late in the afternoon on the final day, during a snowfall and a great thunderstorm, he momentarily opened his eyes, lifted his right hand, and clenched it into a fist. When his hand fell back from this effort, Beethoven was dead."

Ludwig van Beethoven has become for me one of the greatest exemplars of dharma. His courageous struggle with his vocation shows us the precise relationship between the salvation of the individual soul and the salvation of the world.

If you bring forth what is within you, it will save you.

Now we can add a codicil: *If you bring forth what is within you, it will save the world.*

PART V

The Fourth Pillar: "Turn It Over to God"

From the very beginning of our story, Krishna has been teaching Arjuna about action; about making decisions; about hard choices. Do I fight? Do I not fight? Do I act at all? At the outset of their dialogue, Krishna produces a stunning little gem of wisdom for his student (and here again I paraphrase):

"Arjuna, *you do not know how to act because you do not know who you are.*"

You do not know who you are.

Arjuna does not quite get this the first time around.

But, of course, Krishna persists. He teaches that our decisions about our actions flow inexorably from our understanding of who we are. And if we do not know who we are, we will make poor choices.

Krishna plays this theme softly at first. But it will gain in volume through the course of the dialogue, until it reaches a crescendo in the psychedelic theophany of Chapter Eleven.

Krishna knows that he must help Arjuna—and the reader—move toward a clear understanding of his True Nature. And he knows that only this knowledge will allow Arjuna to make wise choices.

"Arjuna," he says, in effect, "we have a Divine nature that we only faintly recognize. Our true nature is unborn, undying, unmanifest, inconceivable to the ordinary mind."

Unborn? Undying? What does this really mean? Well, it's not easy to grasp. It means that those aspects of our lives that we take to be our True Self—our personality, our body, our career, our house, our stories—are not our True Self at all. Our True Self is our soul. This soul is immortal, and is not limited to present forms. Our present bodies and personalities are only temporary shelters, fleetingly inhabited by our souls. These ephemeral forms are, alas, short-lived. The True Self, however, is immortal. It cannot be destroyed.

> [The Self] is not born,
> It does not die;
> Having been,
> It will never not be;
> Unborn, enduring,
> Constant, and primordial,
> It is not killed
> When the body is killed.

This is really quite a speech. But its import is lost on our friend Arjuna.

Krishna gives this teaching several times through the course of the Gita, trying out various metaphors to describe the difference between our *apparent self* and our *True Self*—hoping to find the image that connects. The metaphor that I have found most helpful is the classic "wave" metaphor (which is often cited in other yogic texts, though not explicitly in the Gita). The self (and here we mean the small "s" self, which is our current form and personality) is described as a wave. We're all familiar with the action of the wave: The wave rises in the sea, and having arisen *appears* to have its own form, to be a "thing in itself." In fact, however, the wave is always and everywhere *one with the sea*. It arises from and returns to the sea. It is made of the same stuff as the sea. It *is* the sea in every way. Indeed, even in the fullness of its apparent individual being—its apparent individual "wave-ness"—it is never really *other* than the sea.

Krishna teaches Arjuna an enduring view of the self taken directly from the Vedantic stream of yoga philosophy. In this view, all individual souls (or *atman*) are one with the Ground of Being (or Brahman). Because we are One with the great sea of being, we are all just a single soul, "One without a second." Our True Nature is identical to the nature of Brahman: *sat-chit-ananda,* or being-consciousness-bliss.

Human beings throughout the ages have spent their lives seeking. But seeking what? Seeking God? Seeking consciousness? Seeking the Truth? Krishna's teaching cuts through this seeking: "We are," he says, "what we seek." *Tat tvan asi:* Thou Art That. You are already That which you seek. It is inside. It is already You. It is a done deal. Call off the search! as one great Hindu scholar has written.

Krishna continues his teaching: "Creatures are unmanifest in origin, manifest in the midst of life, and unmanifest again in the end." Another series of obscure phrases from our friend Krishna. To put them in ordinary words, we could say that we manifest from lifetime to lifetime in particular forms: particular bodies, personalities, stories. But these forms—these lifetimes—are transitory.

This teaching is slippery. Indeed, all of the classic yoga texts declare repeatedly that it is a teaching that really cannot be grasped by the mind at all. But (and yogis all agree on this) it can be *realized.* It can be *known intuitively.* Indeed, each of us has intimations of our True Nature from time to time throughout our lives—moments when we know utterly that we are One with all of life. William Wordsworth, in one of his greatest poems, referred to these moments of knowing as "intimations of immortality." These "intimations" sometimes spontaneously arise in our consciousness in moments of quiet—in moments of contemplation, in meditation, in yoga, or just in sitting on the beach at twilight watching a sunset.

But intimations of immortality can also rise in the midst of our hectic lives. Perhaps we are on the subway during a visit to New York City, and we suddenly (and for no apparent reason) feel One with the whole stream of sweating humanity hurtling with us in the rattling underground rocket toward our destination uptown. Suddenly we have this wonderful moment of knowing our Oneness with all beings.

Or, hiking in the woods, we feel an upwelling of kinship with a deer we encounter quietly grazing in a field. Has this happened to you? We are One with that deer. These moments of "knowing" bring with them a calming intuition that everything is OK. That we can really relax. That we can relinquish our striving. That we *are* that which we seek—that, as many yoga texts declare, we are "born divine."

Arjuna has already had these fleeting experiences of Oneness, as Krishna knows. Indeed, each of us has. But Krishna wants Arjuna to notice something *particular* about these realizations. He wants him to see simply this: When we are living in these brief realizations—even for a few moments—they change how we *act*. They change how we behave. They change the choices we make. Just for these few minutes we're different. We're better. We're our best selves—our True Selves.

I know this to be true from my own experience. Back to the subway analogy for a moment. This is an experience that I actually had recently, and it is still very much alive in my memory. I was in New York City on the subway, and I had one of those moments of Oneness. In that mix of smelly, chaotic humanity on the subway I had a moment of feeling at One with all beings. My heart was full of wonder. Of generosity. Of compassion. I gave up my seat. I prayed for those around me. I knew that in absolutely every way that counted I was exactly like the elderly black woman sitting next to me. I knew that she and I were completely alike inside. When I got off the subway, I gladly dropped a five-dollar bill into the hat of the guy playing the guitar on the platform. In those few moments, I was different. Just for those moments, I was the best version of me. The truest version of me. The power of this moment evaporates quickly, of course. I got off the subway and was off about my business in Manhattan. I probably passed by the next subway musician without a thought. But the moment of awakening left behind a trace of something—a trace of knowing.

Have you had an experience like this? In these moments of Oneness, we often feel as if we had dropped in from outer space, and just for a moment are inhabiting our *real* lives. These are moments of waking up from the dream of separation in which we ordinarily live.

If you've had such an experience, you know for a fact that these little awakenings change the way we act. And they highlight the troubling fact that most of the time we live in *exile* from our True Selves.

You do not know how to act, because you do not know who you are.

—— 2 ——

So, Krishna tells Arjuna that his most perilous problem is that *he has forgotten who he is.* Do you relate to this? I think it's one of Krishna's best metaphors.

Often throughout the course of his teaching in the Gita, Krishna will refer to "the brokenness of our memory." "From broken memory understanding is lost," he says, "and from loss of understanding, [we are] ruined." *Ruined!*

This is a central view of the dilemma of the human being in the yoga tradition: We are "wanderers" moving from lifetime to lifetime. Asleep. When we die—when we leave this particular form—we momentarily wake up. We are momentarily rejoined with the Ground of Being. But when we take birth again, we forget. Wordsworth, in his "Ode: Intimations of Immortality", states the case with vivid images:

> Our birth is but a sleep and a forgetting:
> The Soul that rises with us, our life's Star,
> Hath had elsewhere its setting,
> And cometh from afar:
> Not in entire forgetfulness,
> And not in utter nakedness,
> But trailing clouds of glory do we come
> From God, who is our home:
> Heaven lies about us in our infancy.

In the yogic view, as in Wordsworth's, it's through *remembering who we really are* that we are liberated. The transformation of the self is not about adding anything. It is about finding what was already there. In the epigraph of her fine commentary on the Bhagavad Gita, Columbia University scholar Barbara Stoler Miller appropriately quotes T. S. Eliot's lines on memory from *The Four Quartets.*

> This is the use of memory:
> For liberation—not less of love but expanding

Of love beyond desire, and so liberation
From the future as well as the past.

These lines from Eliot might have come directly from the Bhagavad Gita. In remembering who we really are, we are liberated from our striving to be somewhere else, to be someone else. Knowing who we really are liberates us from both the *past*—our overidentification with past experiences of form—and from the *future,* our hopes and fears about future forms.

At the end of the Gita, Arjuna declares:

Krishna, my delusion is destroyed,
and by your grace I have regained memory

I have regained memory. I know who I am. By the end of the story, Arjuna will have been restored to the direct, immediate knowledge of who he is. Then his choices about action will be utterly clear. *You will know how to act when you know who you are.*

— 3 —

About halfway through his dialogue with Krishna, Arjuna begins to get it. And as his eyes open, he sees that Krishna, his friend and charioteer, is not just an ordinary guy. He is much more than a charioteer. To his astonishment, Arjuna begins to see that all along he has been in the presence of a Divine Being. Egad! Krishna is God!!

Upon recognition of Krishna's True Nature, Arjuna has a wonderful and very human moment. He is embarrassed. He says to Krishna: "Sometimes, because we were friends, I rashly said, 'Oh, Krishna!' or, 'Say, friend!'—casual, careless remarks. Whatever I may have said lightly, whether we were playing or resting, alone or in company, sitting together or eating, if it was disrespectful, forgive me for it, O Krishna. I did not know the greatness of your nature, unchanging and imperishable."

This moment endears us to our warrior friend. Arjuna says, in effect, "Gosh, God, I have not been paying you the proper respect." Krishna will later explain to Arjuna that they have been friends through count-

less lives—that they have known and loved each other through the rise
and fall of many forms. Arjuna has forgotten the details, of course, but
he realizes that it is indeed so. Step by step, Krishna has led Arjuna to
understand his life—has led him to understand who he is, who he has
been, and what his pilgrimage across the ages has been like.

Arjuna is now on fire with his love for Krishna. Out of his enthusiasm, he makes a somewhat premature request. He says, "I want to know
you even more." He begs to see Krishna's divine form. "Just as you have
described your infinite glory, O Lord, now I long to see it. I want to see
you as the supreme ruler of creation. O Lord, master of yoga, if you
think me strong enough to behold it, show me your immortal Self."

Of course, Arjuna really doesn't know what he's asking for. But
Krishna wants to grant his wish. He wants to give him full knowledge of
his Divine Self. But because he knows that Arjuna does not really yet
have the capacity to perceive his illumined form, Krishna gives Arjuna
"spiritual vision" to perceive what has previously been outside Arjuna's
limited perceptual range.

What emerges now is one of the great theophanies in all spiritual
writing. The narrator, Sanjaya, recounts what Arjuna sees. It is one of the
most masterful descriptions of the indescribable in all of world literature. (Robert Oppenheimer famously quoted it in 1945, when he was
reaching for words to describe the first controlled explosion of the
atomic bomb over the desert in New Mexico.)

Krishna's divine form, says Sanjaya, "appeared with an infinite
number of faces, ornamented by heavenly jewels, displaying unending
miracles and the countless weapons of his power. Clothed in celestial
garments and covered with garlands, sweet-smelling with heavenly fra-
grances, he showed himself as the infinite Lord, the source of all won-
ders, whose face is everywhere."

Sanjaya continues: "If a thousand suns were to rise in the heavens at
the same time, the blaze of their light would resemble the splendor of
that supreme spirit. There within the body of the God of gods, Arjuna
saw all the manifold forms of the universe united as one. Filled with
amazement, his hair standing on end in ecstasy, he bowed before the
Lord with joined palms . . ."

What is the lesson here for Arjuna? Arjuna—now with "spiritual vision"—perceives the whole world, the entire cosmos, within the Divine form of Krishna. Krishna had already taught Arjuna that awakened ones see the Self in themselves and in all creatures. Now this teaching had become very concrete indeed.

—— 4 ——

Enough! Cries an overwhelmed Arjuna. He soon tells Krishna to take away the vision. The blinding light is too much for his senses to bear. He feels his mortal form being ripped apart by its intensity. Indeed, his consciousness *has* been ripped apart. As we shall see, the vision will change Arjuna. He has received the great teaching: The whole world is within each one of us.

Once Arjuna has regained his equilibrium, Krishna drives home the point: "Arjuna," he says (and I paraphrase), "the explosion of energy and consciousness you have just beheld is also within you. Coiled and ready. Thou Art That. If only you would connect with it. You saw all beings in me. All beings are also in you."

Krishna continues, and says, in effect: "Now seeing the whole picture, you have the information you need in order to make your decisions about how to act in this world. You now know, incontrovertibly, that the whole world is in every being. You have now seen that you are One with it all. You have seen that the whole world is one family. There is no true separation between beings. This is the Truth."

Arjuna is stunned. Humbled. And more than a little freaked out. He wants to hold on to the Truth. But he also wants to turn away from it. "When I'm in the presence of this Truth" he says, haltingly, "I *know* my real nature; and I act accordingly. My actions in such a case are effortlessly noble. But I forget. I forget who I am. Krishna, help! How do I maintain the fragile connection with this Truth?"

Now Krishna gives him the keystone: "Arjuna, that is why I have given you your dharma," he says (and here and in the following paragraphs, I paraphrase Krishna). "Your dharma is your way of staying connected with your True Nature. It is the particular way in which you can devote your life to the welfare of all beings. Your dharma is your very own way of expressing the Truth. Your dharma is the one place where you can penetrate the fleeting world of form. Where you can live as I live, fully connected with the whole world of mind and matter. Where you can live in the sure knowledge that you are not the Doer, but only a vehicle of the great Doer."

Krishna reiterates his earlier teaching: Know your dharma. Do it with all your passion. Let go of the fruits. And now he adds a fourth and final teaching: *And turn it over to me.* Surrender the whole process to me. Surrender your life's work to God—to the divine within you, and to the divine within all beings. In this way your forgetfulness and delusion will slowly disappear. When you are immersed in your dharma, the wave becomes the sea again. Don't you see? Dharma is your path home.

"Now do you see?" says Krishna. "In this mortal life you must *walk by faith*. You must walk by faith, not by the sight of your limited human vision. In order to walk by faith, you must gradually learn to trust me and my guidance. You must gradually learn to surrender your will. You cannot steer your dharma with the vehicle of self-will—the will of the small "s" self. Self-will will always steer you toward delusion, toward forgetfulness, toward separation. This self-will—driven by the grasping of small "s" self—is the greatest enemy of freedom and Oneness."

Krishna's teaching at this point in the dialogue becomes bold and challenging: "Keep all your senses tuned to the ineffable at all times. Listen for and follow my guidance every step of the way. Let go of doubt. And finally, see Me in every human being. See the Divine within yourself. Within everyone. And act accordingly. Your actions will be effortlessly noble—and will create happiness for you and for the whole world."

Arjuna now understands that the real task he must master in this lifetime is *learning to walk by faith*. And he realizes that enacting his dharma is, in itself, the greatest act of faith.

In this final section of the book, then, we will explore two of the central themes in Krishna's powerful final lessons to Arjuna:

1. Walk by faith.
2. Take yourself to zero.

We will examine the lives of two great examplars of these principles—beginning with an investigation of the astonishing life of Harriet Tubman, a nineteenth-century American slave who surrendered her life into the hands of God, and who discovered, as Thoreau did, that one person's freedom could burst the fetters off a million slaves. And finally, we'll look at the life of Mohandas K. Gandhi, perhaps history's most brilliant student and exemplar of the Bhagavad Gita. In the process, we will also revisit the stories of our old friends Brian (the priest) and Katherine (the dean) as they continue to come to grips with the perils and promise of their own individual dharmas.

ELEVEN

Harriet Tubman: Walk by Faith

Most families have dharma teaching-stories. Of course we don't call them that. But think for a moment of your own family's dharma stories. These are usually tales of the courage and character of some colorful forebear, who against big odds thrived in her authentic calling. When these tales are told over and over again they develop a flavor of myth. The young people at the grown-ups' table on Thanksgiving roll their eyes when they hear them for the twentieth time. Still, these stories creep into our psyches, and help to form our sense of what might be possible for us.

In my own family, my grandmother, Armeda Van Demark Crothers, was the teller of these tales. She told them at Sunday dinner, or seated in a wicker rocking chair on the front porch of the family summer cottage. One of her favorites was the story of my great-great-great grandfather, Dr. Elias Willard Frisbie. Dr. Frisbie lived from 1799 until 1860 in the little town of Phelps, New York—the upstate village where I spent happy weeks and months as a kid, and where my grandmother lived out her entire life.

Elias Frisbie was an ardent abolitionist, and his house was a hub on the so-called "Underground Railroad" during the decade leading up to the Civil War. The Underground Railroad—as every tenth-grader in Phelps knows—provided a network of invisible support to fugitive slaves from the Deep South all the way to Canada. My grandmother told stories of Dr. Frisbie's risky commitment to this invisible road to freedom, and of his involvement with fugitive slave Harriet Tubman, whose own home was in the nearby village of Auburn, New York. Grandma emphasized: By helping runaway slaves, Dr. Frisbie put himself in serious danger. His actions were in direct violation of the Fugitive Slave Law of 1850.

Grandma knew great dharma material when she heard it. She told tales of the midnight movement of fugitive black faces through the woods around Phelps; of near encounters with police; of the dreaded slave catchers who occasionally haunted the little village and surreptitiously surveilled suspect homes. Her tale usually ended with the story of a triumphant parade in Phelps—a parade of slaves and their white supporters—that went right up the center of town. Dr. Frisbie was at its head. And the moral of the story? Do what you know is right even if you have to take risks. The fine Dr. Frisbie was hewing to his high ideals.

Grandma's story worked its intended magic. Dr. Frisbie—and Harriet Tubman and her network of freedom fighters—captured my imagination. And the lesson I took from the story could have come from Krishna himself: A guy has got to do what a guy has got to do.

As I've grown older, I've become intrigued with Elias Frisbie's interactions with the near-mythic figure of Harriet Tubman. Grandma didn't know enough about Frisbie's relationship with Tubman to include the details in her official story, but I've learned as much as I can about them, and I now weave these nuggets into the original story when I tell it to my nieces and nephews. This, I suppose, is how a family's dharma story evolves.

—— 2 ——

Harriet Tubman—a diminutive, unprepossessing, and mammothly determined fugitive slave—was the most famous rescuer of slaves in the American South in the decade between 1850 and 1860. She carried out a string of at least nineteen daring raids into slaveholding territories—leading her enslaved family and friends (and practically anyone who dared to come) out of bondage in the South and all the way to freedom in Canada. Her hair-raising journeys became the stuff of legend—and were made more notorious by the fact that Tubman was herself a fugitive slave and subject at any time to recapture and the horror of reenslavement. (Actually, Tubman would most likely not have been reenslaved had she been caught. She would have just been hung. By the time the Civil War erupted there was a price of $40,000 on her head—and she was hated and feared by Southern slave owners.)

Stories of Tubman's raids into the South are toe curling. By all accounts, she had an uncanny ability to evade danger. She could evaporate into thin air with a whole troop of fugitives (and she sometimes led as many as ten or twelve out at a time). She had a second sense about when to move and when to stay under cover—hunches that often defied common sense. She had an unerring sense of which riverbank to follow, which house might be safe, which house might harbor danger. There are edge-of-your-seat accounts of her accidentally coming face-to-face with former masters during her forays south—once on the very plantation from which she had herself escaped. These stories always end with her avoiding recognition through some clever spur-of-the moment disguise: pulling a bonnet down over her face, or putting her nose in a newspaper (though she could not read a word).

When one drills down into these tales, one finds that they flesh out in vivid fashion one critical component of dharma: the issue of "guidance." Harriet was widely believed to have been guided directly by God—called by him, and guided by him every step of the way. Within months of her near-miraculous escape from a plantation in Maryland, she had the distinct sense of a call, a voice inside that said, "Harriet Tubman, I want you to help free others." Tubman answered back to God, "Find somebody else. Can't do it. You kidding?"

The stories of a "call" such as Harriet received are omnipresent in the spiritual and religious world: Jonah and the whale, Moses in Egypt, St. Paul on the road to Damascus. "The Call" is an archetype of the spiritual imagination. It is nothing less than the call to be absolutely yourself.

The call to Harriet was repeated over and over again—as it has to be in these stories, since the first response is always "no." Of course, in this particular story Tubman finally said yes, but very reluctantly. Doubt and indecision are always a central aspect of "call" stories, and Arjuna is our antiheroic example. Harriet decided that if she were going to respond to this nagging call, she would have to put herself in God's hands, because she had no idea how to pull it off by herself. "If you've called me to this, Lord, then you'll damn sure have to do it, 'cause I can't."

Harriet followed her guidance. She prayed. She listened. And she found the guidance she received stunningly reliable. Eventually, Harriet learned to walk by faith, not by sight. And her faith was, apparently, contagious, for everyone else began to trust her as well. Fugitives whom she helped free soon enough learned: If she says go, go. If she says stay, stay.

A moment-by-moment trust in Divine guidance is central to Krishna's teaching. He teaches: "To know when to act and when to refrain from action, what is right action and what is wrong, what brings security and what brings insecurity, what brings freedom and what brings bondage: These are the signs of a pure mind."

To know when to act, and when not to act.

Harriet Tubman's dharma story allows us to examine the question of guidance. How does Divine guidance actually work? Is there really such a thing? Is it from God, or is it from an ineffable Inner Self? Is it available even to us?

— 3 —

Harriet Tubman was born into slavery in 1825. (Her mother had arrived on a slave ship directly from Africa, and was bought by a Maryland family named Pattison.) As a girl, Harriet learned the central facts of slavery: Your body is not your own, your life is not your own, your labor is not your own, and your family is not your own. This last fact was a source of particular suffering for young Harriet. She learned early on that your kin can be sold "downriver" at any moment, and you have absolutely no recourse. Once sold, families were rarely reunited. Tubman watched as her mother's family—sisters and brothers—were auctioned off in front of her, while the family stood by in horror and agony.

How would one manage the violence and powerlessness of such a life? Harriet's mother managed it by developing a sustaining faith in God, and she taught this faith to Harriet. The entire family was illiterate, so they never actually read the Bible, but they learned Bible stories by heart—especially the Old Testament stories of the suffering of God's people in Egypt, and their eventual escape into the Promised Land. These stories were made vivid in Harriet's imagination in chants sung rhythmically while at work in the fields, and in stories told at night huddled together in the slave cabin.

Harriet would need every ounce of her mother's faith: When she was only five years old, a "Miss Susan" drove up to Pattison's plantation and asked for a young girl to take care of a baby. Pattison sent Harriet off with "Miss Susan" that very instant—to a new and harrowing home far from her parents. This experience of sudden exile was repeated over and over again throughout Harriet's childhood. By the time she was fifteen she had had many masters, though she eventually ended up back at Pattison's. She said later, "I grew up like a neglected weed—ignorant of liberty, having no experience of it."

By the time she was in her teens, Tubman had become a field hand which she vastly preferred to being a house slave. In the fields, she developed physical and mental stamina, and enjoyed the taste of the personal power this brought her. Outdoors—where she was not so directly under the shoe of the master—she began to get a taste of freedom. She wanted more.

In 1849, Harriet learned quite by accident that for the previous decade she and her family had been held illegally in slavery, for they had—unbeknownst to them—actually been freed by Master Pattison's will at his death ten years earlier. Pattison's heir had conveniently neglected to inform them of this. The discovery of this outrageous betrayal made Harriet blind with rage. What to do? She turned first to her faith. She decided to begin a prayer vigil for the soul of her master (Pattison's heir), whom she now knew to be a charlatan of the worst sort. She prayed fervently that his heart would be changed.

His heart was not changed. But Harriet's was. Tubman learned a lesson: She saw that she would have to take an active role in God's plan for her. She could no longer be only a passive supplicant. She needed to learn to skillfully combine *prayer and action*—a most Gita-like insight.

Harriet came to believe that she had a moral duty to free herself. She had not only a *right* but a *duty* to be free: "I had reasoned this out in my mind," she said later. "There was one of two things I had a right to, liberty or death; if I could not have one I would have the other."

For years before her escape, Harriet had recurring dreams of her flight to freedom. In the dream, she was "flying over fields and towns, and rivers and mountains, looking down upon them 'like a bird,' and reaching at last a great fence, or sometimes a river, over which she would try to fly . . . "It 'peared like I wouldn't have the strength, and just as I was sinkin' down, there would be ladies all drest in white over there, and they would put out their arms and pull me 'cross.' "

This dream of flight to freedom was, of course, a central theme in African American spirituality, and often included the image of a river (usually the River Jordan) and visions of crossing that river—or of ascending into Heaven. Freedom and death were closely linked in the spiritual imagination of slaves. Their songs were filled with these images:

> I looked over Jordan, and what did I see?
> Coming for to carry me home,
> A band of angels coming after me,
> Coming for to carry me home.

When Harriet was twenty-seven, she learned that her master intended to put her up for auction. This was the last straw. She decided to make her move. It appears that Harriet planned her escape very methodically, and then quietly slipped away from her master's estate on September 24, 1850. She was immediately pursued by slave catchers.

Harriet's escape was extraordinary by any measure. Most fugitive slaves were men, but Harriet was a woman still in her twenties. She had never been out of her home county. She knew no more than most slaves did about the path to freedom. She knew only a few pieces of slave lore: She knew to move at night, she knew to follow the riverbanks leading north, and she knew to follow the North Star. She had often heard the song filled with clues about the route to freedom: "Follow the Drinkin' Gourd." The drinking gourd referred, of course, to the constellation we call The Big Dipper—whose two end-stars point to the North Star.

When the sun come back and the quail calls,
Follow the drinkin' gourd.
For the old man a-waitin' to carry you to freedom
If you follow the drinkin' gourd.

The riverbank make a very good road.
The dead trees show you the way.
Left foot, right foot, travel on,
Follow the drinkin' gourd

There's another river on the other side,
Follow the drinkin' gourd.
When the great river meets the little river there,
Follow the drinkin' gourd

One can only imagine the terror of this young woman as she tore stealthily through the brush and woods of nighttime Maryland—the sound of bloodhounds baying in pursuit. She had a price on her head: On October 3, the *Cambridge Democrat* newspaper published a runaway slave notice: "MINTY, aged about 27 years, is of a chestnut color, fine looking and bout 5 feet high." (Tubman's birth name was Araminta: thus, MINTY.) Readers were advised that Minty would fetch $50 if she were captured in Maryland, or $100 if she were found out of the state.

By her own accounting, Harriet's long journey out of the Maryland/Delaware peninsula was done entirely on foot—moving northeast along the Choptank River. ("The riverbank make a very good road.") It's most likely that she then received help from Quakers in the region—and it's almost certain that she made contact with members of the already-formed Underground Railroad, who helped her find her way to Philadelphia.

Philadelphia was, of course, the city of brotherly love. It was a promised land for fugitive slaves, and a mecca for black reformers. Harriet settled in to her newly adopted city as best she could. She was free, yes. But she was also penniless, and in constant peril of recapture.

—— 4 ——

The second act of this drama comes almost immediately on the heels of the first. In late 1850, after a number of months of freedom in Philadelphia, Harriet got word from Maryland that her niece, Kizzy, was about to be "sold downriver" into the Deep South—precisely the way Tubman's sister had been many years before. This was a fork in the road for Harriet. She decided that she must put her own freedom on the line to help rescue her niece. She must go back into Maryland—a slave state where she herself was wanted as a fugitive—to help with the rescue.

Harriet did not make this decision lightly. She was awash in doubt and fear—and terrified at the prospect of recapture. But she knew that she had to act in spite of the fear. Tubman realized that her fate was tied together with that of her family and indeed that of her whole people. She came to understand that she could not have freedom just for herself. Her entire race was at risk if any one of its members was enslaved. At this point, Harriet's own personal journey to freedom expanded vastly to include the potential freedom of her whole people. She decided that she would let herself be used by this great work.

Very little is known about Tubman's rescue of Kizzy. It appears that Harriet's brothers in Maryland assisted effectively in the abduction— and that Kizzy narrowly escaped the slave auction by days or even hours. Astonishingly, Tubman was able to navigate the completely alien streets of Baltimore. She managed to locate help, find a safe house, and eventually guide Kizzy to freedom with her in Philadelphia.

The success of her first rescue lit Harriet's dharma fire. She now felt her calling intensely. She made a second trip in 1851, and on this trip rescued one of her brothers and two other friends. By this time, she had begun to make strong connections within the network of the Underground Railroad. She slowly began to master the abductor's art: evasion, disguise, secret underground channels, forests, and riverbanks. She would become very familiar indeed with the drinking gourd.

Tubman now got to know the network of thousands of white abolitionists like Elias Frisbie who were willing to put their own safety on the line for her. This silent, intrepid volunteer army had developed a network of "stations" or "depots"—a clandestine network designed to support the movement of fugitive slaves all the way from the Deep South to freedom in the North. The network included so-called "stationmasters," "conductors," and elaborate transportation schemes for "cargo." "Depots" could be hidden rooms in basements, like Dr. Frisbie's, or hideaways in attics, barns, potato cellars, even caves. There were secret tunnels and fake closets. Fugitives were transported alive in coffins, crates, and barrels.

Most conductors on the Underground Railroad only conveyed slaves from one depot to the next, and they often knew little about the full extent of the network. The less they knew, perhaps, the better. There were, however, a few heroic "abductors" who ventured deep into the slave states to personally extract slaves. Tubman was one of these. Almost all of the rest were white men. But then there was Harriet Tubman: a small, quiet, uneducated woman—but a force of nature. Or we might better say, a force of dharma. Her reputation eventually eclipsed all the others'.

Harriet slowly began to dedicate her entire life to this work. She made at least one trip a year—sometimes two—deep into slave territory. She often rescued at least ten fugitives at a time. She kept to the back roads and never traveled by day. She always made her trips in the winter, when the nights were long and dark. Eventually, Tubman decided that Canada was the new Canaan. "I wouldn't trust Uncle Sam with my people no longer," she said, "but I brought 'em clear off to Canada."

Astonishingly, the funds for Tubman's trips came almost entirely from her own work as a cook and a domestic. She worked to save money during the spring and summer, and then during the fall, she would plan her trips—carrying them out when the nights became longest.

— 5 —

Tubman came to believe that she would be guided by God at every step along the way. The images she used in talking about her "journeys" were saturated with spiritual archetypes. She used bible stories of the Exodus to create a context for her journeys. She used the great spirituals as cues for "troops" to move or stay put, to show themselves or hide themselves away. She prayed regularly with her fugitives. Though as we've seen, Harriet was illiterate, nonetheless she could quote extensively and accurately from the Bible, and was keenly aware of the significance of characters and incidents from both the Old and the New Testament.

Harriet Tubman was widely believed to be protected by angels. Over the years, an air of mystery and awe began to grow up around her. Said fellow abductor Thomas Garrett, "Harriet seems to have a special angel to guard her on her journey of mercy . . . and confidence that God will preserve her from harm in all her perilous journeys."

Most of the really dramatic accounts of Harriet's "guidance" came from others—not from Harriet herself, who was remarkably quiet about her methods. Garrett said, "I never met with any person of any color who had more confidence in the voice of God, as spoken direct to her soul."

Harriet's so-called "second sight"—her reliance on guidance—would become legendary among fugitives, and among the network of conductors and stationmasters on the Underground Railroad. Fugitive slaves whom she freed later told remarkable stories about their adventures with her. In the midst of a flight, Harriet would suddenly insist that the troop of fugitives stop and hide themselves away. Then she would start out again in an entirely new direction. Later, they would discover that they had narrowly escaped capture. Tubman said about these moments, "When danger is near, it appears like my heart goes flutter, flutter." She told a friend that she believed that her uncanny "second sight" was a gift that she inherited from her father, who was apparently known for prophecies and guidance.

Her biographer, Catherine Clinton, gives us a classic Tubman story: "During one trip aboard a boat, a ticket collector asked Harriet and her companion, a fugitive named Tilly, to step aside while he took others' tickets. Tilly was wild with fear, but Tubman kept calm and prayed, 'Oh, Lord, you have been with me in six troubles, don't desert me in the seventh.' She kept murmuring prayers, and to Tilly's great surprise, the incantation worked: The ticket collector let them proceed, and they made it to their destination without further interference."

It was fitting that Tubman came to be called "Moses," for the Old Testament Moses underwent remarkably similar trials, and the Moses story is likewise full of conflicts between doubt and faith, and eventual reliance on God's usually inconvenient will.

How, precisely, does this experience of guidance work? The great seventeenth-century Jesuit writer, Jean-Pierre de Caussade, speaks directly to this question in his spiritual classic *Abandonment to Divine Providence*:

> "When God becomes our guide he insists that we trust him without reservations and put aside all nervousness about his guidance. We are sent along the path he has chosen for us, but we cannot see it, and nothing we have read is any help to us. Were we acting on our own we should have to rely on our experience. It would be too risky to do anything else. But it is very different when God acts with us. Divine action is always new and fresh, it never retraces its steps, but always finds new routes."

Divine action is always new and fresh. This is a startlingly accurate insight by de Caussade. Responding to the "freshness" of divine guidance requires a certain docility of the will, flexibility, and a kind of radical trust. This trust is particularly required, because, as de Caussade says frequently, when we are led by the spirit, the guidance we receive is often shrouded in darkness. Krishna grasped this same point. He says to Arjuna: "These actions are enveloped in smoke."

The yoga tradition is full of teaching stories about divine guidance, and in these stories, sure enough, this guidance is always enshrouded in darkness, in "a cloud," or in "smoke." In one of the greatest of these yoga tales—told in countless versions—a pilgrim is on an important journey. He travels only at night, and carries a lantern, but the lantern only illuminates the path just a few feet ahead of him. He knows that this slim illumination is all he needs. He does not need to see the whole path ahead. He trusts that he can make the entire journey seeing only the immediate next steps.

De Caussade picks up the theme: "When we are led by this action, we have no idea where we are going, for the paths we tread cannot be discovered from books or by any of our thoughts. But these paths are always opened in front of us and we are impelled along them. Imagine we are in a strange district at night and are crossing fields unmarked by any path, but we have a guide. He asks no advice nor tells us of his plans. So what can we do except trust him? It is no use trying to see where we are, look at maps or question passersby. That would not be tolerated by a guide who wants us to rely on him. He will get satisfaction from overcoming our fears and doubts, and will insist that we have complete trust in him."

One of the most difficult aspects of faith is the *suspension of one's own preconceived ideas* about how to proceed. The willing suspension of preconceived plans and schemes is absolutely required, as Harriet Tubman discovered. These plans—*our* plans—are then gradually replaced by a growing trust in moment-by-moment guidance.

Harriet's trips were characterized by this very "shroud of darkness," and also by stunning acts of creativity all along the way. When Harriet and her current band of fugitives finally reached the suspension bridge that led her party across the Niagara into Canada, she would routinely lead the party in songs of thanksgiving, great spirituals, and hymns of praise. She understood that a successful trip was not her doing. She saw clearly that she was "not the Doer." Thanks should be given!

— 6 —

Remember our friend Brian the priest? When last we left him, he was on the floor of his own particular chariot. He was, you will recall, caught in long-standing inner conflict: Should he make a belated choice for what he knew was his true calling as a church musician? Or should he remain in the now-familiar role of rector of his small parish church? It was not a black-or-white choice by any means, as you will recall. He was in many ways well suited to the role of rector. He knew that he was being useful in the role. His family was proud of him. But his deepest aspirations had not been realized. He felt empty, dissatisfied, and deeply afraid he would die without having fully lived. Brian had lived with a quiet sense of self-betrayal for twenty years. As he reached his forty-fifth year, he could begin to see that his life would at some point end. And he wondered more and more frequently: Is there still time for me to be who I really am?

Around the time of his forty-fifth birthday, Brian became seriously depressed. He was paralyzed—like Arjuna—in the face of two courses of action, both of which now seemed difficult. The more he thought about it, the more impossible the situation seemed. He became more and more paralyzed. He started to drink heavily.

Finally, out of desperation, Brian did something very wise. He requested a leave of absence from his post as rector. His depression was his "second sense" kicking in. Something in him simply refused to go on. This refusal was a wise inner move: When you are enveloped in doubt, it is sometimes best just to stop. When in doubt don't! Instead of moving forward in a daze, can you allow yourself to stop and experience the pain of the doubt? Can you investigate the doubt itself? This is precisely what Arjuna had to do. The entire dialogue of the Gita happens in a kind of "time-out" for Arjuna, as he explores his doubt. All forward movement is suspended, and an intense inquiry takes place.

"Suspending forward movement" was not that easy for Brian. The bishop had a shortage of good priests upon whom to call, and he was not pleased to let Brian go. The bishop, like Brian's mother, wrote Brian's doubts off as a midlife crisis. "Priests have these crises of faith," said the bishop. "He'll get through it."

In spite of the resistance, Brian entered into a time of inquiry. This was itself a pivotal act of faith. Sometimes just stopping can be the act that allows the solution to emerge. Brian spent three months at a Jesuit retreat center. I had given him de Caussade's *Abandonment to Divine Providence* before he left, and also one of my old copies of the Gita.

I visited with Brian after he had been at the retreat center for a month. We had lunch together in the refectory. He'd been studying de Caussade's book, and he'd vigorously underlined this passage in it: "Now it is surely obvious that the only way to receive [guidance] is to put oneself quietly in the hands of God, and that none of our own efforts and mental striving can be of any use at all."

None of our own efforts and mental striving can be of any use at all. At all? Brian had come to feel the wearying truth of this.

De Caussade nails this point: "This work in our souls cannot be accomplished by cleverness, intelligence, or any subtlety of mind, but only by completely abandoning ourselves to the divine action, becoming like metal poured into a mold, or a canvas waiting for the brush, or marble under the sculptor's hands."

Brian had to surrender his will. He had to be willing to do what he was called to do. And he had to put *everything* on the table. Nothing held back. This meant that he had to be willing to continue being rector if that was the guidance he received, and he had to be willing to bring everything he had even to that vocation.

Several weeks into his retreat, Brian made another smart move: He entered into a relationship with an old priest/confessor at the center. (Notice once again what a pivotal role mentors play in dharma decisions.) Father Bede had been a monk for forty years, and he was now the chief spiritual director at the retreat. Bede was sanguine about Brian's situation, but forceful. He gave Brian the same message repeatedly: "For the sake of God, boy, let go of all this obsessive worry and fretting. You are powerless over such a mess." Bede had faith that Brian would be guided. And Brian, who had much less faith, was able to hitchhike on Bede's. Slowly, and as a result of pure desperation, Brian began to loosen his grip on the outcome.

Brian and I talked about his process that day at lunch. I was caught up in the writing of this book, and was fascinated by questions of divine guidance. I was curious: How do you know the will of God? And when you do *think* you know it, *how can you be certain that it's not just your own will in disguise?* During lunch that day, Brian and I put together a list of how the process seems to work.

1. First of all, "ask for guidance." As it turns out, this is remarkably important, and it's something most of us almost always forget to do. It seems that there is something about *actually asking* that jump-starts a process. And sometimes asking repeatedly is required. Even begging.

2. Then (something else we usually forget) "listen for the response." It helps, says Bede, to "actively listen." To turn over every stone in your search for clues to the response. These responses usually come in subtle ways—through hunches, fleeting images, intuitions. Do you think this is all hooey? That skepticism is OK, said Bede. Even healthy. But listen anyway. Allow yourself to be surprised.

3. Next (another good principle from Bede), "When you get a response, check it out." Check it out with friends, with mentors. Talk about it. This, says Bede, is a classic principle of guidance: Test the guidance.

Real guidance will stand up to sustained testing. False guidance—which is usually just our own will trying to have its way—will not stand up to ongoing scrutiny.

4. Next comes a principle that I've discovered in my own life: "Once you *do* begin to get clarity, wait to act until you have at least a kernel of inner certitude." *Wait to act.* One thing I've learned for sure after a bunch of ham-handed decisions to act is that one almost never regrets slowing things down. We often *do,* however, regret speeding things up. Important decisions very often cannot be hurried. This is wonderfully exemplified by Arjuna, whose chief courage in the pages of the Gita is shown through his willingness to slow down the action and investigate deliberately and relentlessly. Note: Arjuna, the quintessential man of action, spends the entire Gita on his butt.

5. Once there is "a flavor of certitude," says Bede, then "pray for the courage to take action." It's not uncommon for us to get to certitude and then realize that we don't really *want* to take the action. We're not willing. Or we don't have the courage. Or it's too inconvenient. Here's an important Bede tip: You can pray for the *willingness.* You can pray for the courage. You can pray for absolutely everything you need along the way.

6. Bede suggests a corollary to #5, and this is a suggestion that both Brian and I really liked: "Let go of the attempt to eliminate risk from these decisions and actions." The presence of a sense of risk is only an indication that you're at an important crossroads. Risk cannot be eliminated, and the *attempt* to eliminate it will only lead you back to paralysis. In important dharma decisions, we never get to 100 percent certitude.

7. Next, we agreed: "Move forward methodically." Begin to take action in support of your choice. Taking action at this point is critical to keeping the process moving. You will continue to be guided as you take action. Be aware that you are led by faith and not by sight, and that the whole process may be shrouded in darkness. Learn to feel your way along.

8. And finally, of course, the very central teaching of the Gita: "Let go of the outcome." Let go of any clinging to how this all comes out. You cannot measure your actions at this point by the conventional wisdom about success and failure.

After we had sketched out this list, Brian and I got to talking about the Gita. He'd been reading it, along with de Caussade. He wanted to talk about one of Krishna's speeches in particular that spoke to him. Krishna says: "By fulfilling the obligations he is born with, a person never comes to grief. No one should abandon duties because he sees defects in them. Every action, every activity is surrounded by smoke."

Smoke again.

— 7 —

By the time the Civil War broke out, Harriet Tubman had become the terror of slave owners all over the South. They were desperate to nail her. The great Boston writer and abolitionist Thomas Wentworth Higginson hailed her in his speeches as "a modern-day Joan of Arc," and set her up as the model of noble action. Harriet herself thought this was all bunk, and took little notice.

After the Civil War began, Harriet's career took an interesting turn. She was quietly hired by the Union Army to be a war-time spy. She helped to train and guide a whole cadre of scouts and spies who infiltrated the territory held by the Confederacy—mapping it, and observing the movement of Southern troops. Tubman was listed (confoundingly to many at the time) as a "commander" of her men—and she and her spy ring worked directly under the guidance of the Secretary of War.

In the role of Union spy, Tubman continued to free slaves. Indeed, her raids during the war became even more daring than before, supported as they now were by the entire Union Army. There is one practically mythic—but absolutely true—story of a Tubman sneak attack in the middle of the night on a great plantation in South Carolina. During this attack, she spirited away more than 750 slaves onto a Union gunboat, leaving the estate of the great local plantation humiliated and bereft of slaves. This was classic Tubman: She worked stealthily behind the scenes, and then struck when least expected.

During the Civil War, Harriet was at the peak of her powers. She was hugely creative, in precisely the way de Caussade predicted one would be when led by the spirit. Tubman was constantly coming up with brilliant solutions on the spot—solutions that stunned her comrades. She had no schooling whatsoever in military affairs, so she was not constrained by any concepts about how things *should* be done. She just trusted her own gut. Her motto was always, "Just keep going."

This motto, "Just keep going" is instructive. What I find most important, finally, about the Harriet Tubman story is her particular combination of faith and action. These two qualities reinforce each other. Together they are fire and gasoline. We will explore this more thoroughly in the next chapter of this book, when we look at the life of Mahatma Gandhi. But it's important to note this principle here: *Discerning action strengthens faith.* This is a common thread in all of our stories.

— 8 —

By the end of his three-month retreat, Brian had made his decision. ("Actually," he would correct me, "the decision made me.") "When I really did finally let go," he said, "all hell broke loose. Everything shifted."

Brian and I had not charted this aspect of the process in our lunch. But Brian's story added a new piece: The hardest work comes in getting to the decision. Once the decision is made, it is as if the decision itself lays down some kind of invisible tracks—and the cart of dharma just rolls forward, sometimes at shocking speed. Forget about trying to slow down this part of the process.

Brian's dharma life spilled forward dramatically: It turns out that a position within the national church had just opened up—music director at an innovative program to enliven the sacred music in parishes all over the country. The director of the program just happened to be on retreat at the same time Brian was. They got to know each other, and he saw that Brian was the perfect guy for the job. He recruited Brian at the self-same table where we had worked on our list.

In the five years since Brian's retreat, he has developed the national sacred music institute into a well-functioning organization. He has been creative in the role, and fully engaged. He brings parish music directors (his authentic tribe) to the institute to help inspire and direct them. He founded a summer choir camp. Brian is living his dharma: unified at last.

Several years ago, Brian came back to give a sermon in his old parish, and invited me to come. I noticed in his sermon that he frequently used the archetype of "the journey" when talking to parishioners. He used a passage from Exodus that describes Moses and the journey out of Egypt. He talked about the bondage of inauthenticity—the bondage of the false self, the bondage of self-will. And he talked about the exhilaration of freedom. Those of us who have been in bondage and have made the journey to freedom are particularly touched by the suffering of others who are still in shackles. Remember Thoreau: One authentic act of freedom can knock the fetters from a million slaves.

—— 9 ——

Harriet Tubman returned home a war hero. She would spend the rest of her life helping her African American brothers and sisters regain dignity, respect, and freedom. As you can imagine, this was an uphill battle.

As a harbinger of things to come, even as an exhausted Tubman was returning home from the war on a Northbound passenger train—traveling from Virginia to her home in Auburn, New York—she was the victim of predictable race prejudice. She was violently dragged from her coach seat by a conductor who decided that her papers must have been forged. How could a black woman be legally carrying a soldier's pass? How could she be a "commander"? Harriet was then thrown into the baggage compartment for the remainder of the trip. She would live with this kind of violence for the rest of her life. It did not stop her.

After she returned to Auburn, Harriet focused her mammoth energies on helping the many needy and dispossessed African Americans in her own region of New York. She poured all of her own personal resources into this task—taking many needy folk into her own home. Her dream was to establish a separate charitable institution in Auburn for the neglected of her race. She finally did accomplish this—at the age of eighty-five. She eventually developed the Harriet Tubman Home for the Aged—a home that still exists to serve the community today.

In what spare time she had, Harriet Tubman also became a grand old lady on the suffrage circuit. She was by all accounts a spellbinding speaker at suffrage events. Our friend Susan B. Anthony introduced her as a living legend at the NYS Women's Suffrage Association held in 1904. One local newspaper described the dramatic scene: "The old woman was once a slave and as she stood before the assemblage in her cheap black gown and coat and a big black straw bonnet without adornment, her hand held in Miss Anthony's, she impressed one with the venerable dignity of her appearance." At the same event, Tubman told the rapt crowd, "I was conductor of the Underground Railroad for eight years, and I can say what most conductors can't say—I never ran my train off the track and I never lost a passenger."

Tubman struggled to make ends meet until the end of her life. She was never compensated for her war service (an American scandal that has never been repaired). She gave away everything she had. None of the obstacles she faced ever stopped her for long. She just kept moving forward. She always remembered her refrain on the Underground Railroad: "If you are tired, keep going; if you are scared, keep going; if you are hungry, keep going; if you want to taste freedom, keep going."

Later in life, Tubman's co-abductor Thomas Garrett said something telling about Harriet: "The strangest thing about this woman is, she does not know, or appears not to know, that she has done anything worth notice." This quality is an outward and visible sign of true dharma. One does not seek credit. The credit goes to God—the real Doer. Says Krishna: "Those who follow the path of service, who have completely purified themselves and conquered their senses and self-will, see the Self in all creatures and are untouched by any action they perform. Those who know this truth, whose consciousness is unified, think always, I am not the Doer."

Harriet, indeed, always said that she did not feel she had any special powers whatsoever, just that she was especially blessed. Not unlike Joan of Arc, throughout her life, Tubman viewed herself as an instrument of God. She trusted in the power of prayer, and in the individual's ability to seize her own destiny. She believed that any person who sought to could be guided by God's hand—just as she had been.

"Each and every person has the light of God within," she said.

― TWELVE ―

Mohandas K. Gandhi:
Take Yourself to Zero

On August 16, 1908, more than two thousand Indian nationals living in Transvaal, South Africa, joined at a local Hindu temple to burn their South African registration certificates. They were protesting recently enacted legislation—called the Black Act—that would dramatically limit their civil rights in South Africa. The thousands of Indian men and women who participated in this action were no doubt terrified, fearing the reprisals of the notoriously repressive South African government. And they were also very likely astonished at their own actions that day, and at the fact that they had summoned the courage to take a risky stand against tyranny. Much of their courage issued from the trust they had in their leader and champion in this action. He was a powerful and compelling little Indian barrister whom they had come to love. He was Mohandas K. Gandhi—who would later come to be known as "Mahatma Gandhi," or Great Soul, and who would eventually lead 400 million Indians out of bondage to the British Empire. The protest against the Black Act in South Africa was young Gandhi's first act of mass civil disobedience.

The act of civil disobedience carried out in Transvaal on that August day more than a century ago was more successful than anyone in the Indian community could have hoped. The international press covered the event widely, and compared it to the Boston Tea Party. Gandhi and his fellows had deftly painted the government into a corner—all without violence of any kind. Even Gandhi himself was surprised at the power—he would later call it Soul Force—of this kind of action. What began that day was his development of the art of *satyagraha* (literally, "clinging to truth") that would, over the course of the next two decades, change the face of the world. "Thus came into being," wrote Gandhi much later in his life, "the moral equivalent of war."

Civil disobedience, based on the principles of *satyagraha,* would become a staple of Gandhi's tool kit for the rest of his life, and would be the central pillar of his strategy to end British colonial rule in India. This *satyagraha*—this "clinging to truth"—was an entirely new method of fighting injustice. Instead of fanning hatred with hatred, Gandhi insisted upon returning love for hatred and respect for contempt.

Any exploration of dharma that begins with Henry David Thoreau must end with Mohandas K. Gandhi. These two exemplars of "Soul Force" lived a century apart, but with the perspective of time they increasingly appear as brothers. Thoreau's life and writing—especially his essay *On Civil Disobedience* and his masterpiece, *Walden*—profoundly influenced Gandhi. In many ways, we might say that Gandhi finished what Thoreau started. *Satyagraha* was, after all, the very embodiment of the doctrine of "truth in action" about which Thoreau had written so passionately almost a century earlier.

—— 2 ——

Mohandas K. Gandhi began his adult life as a shy, tongue-tied Indian barrister who failed at most everything he tried. He was plagued by fears and doubts. He was socially inept. At the age of twenty-three, he had left his native India for South Africa—a last attempt to salvage a foundering legal career. (Young Gandhi had become famous in the Indian legal world for once fleeing a courtroom in terror when he had been called upon to present a difficult argument. He later became known as "the briefless barrister," because after this embarrassment no one would give him a case.) Yet when Gandhi returned to India just ten years later, he was hailed as "Mahatma," and quickly became the acknowledged leader of the hundreds of millions of Indian people hungry for self-respect, self-reliance, and independence from Great Britain.

How had this transformation happened? What precisely was Gandhi doing between his ignominious departure from India—tail between his legs—and his triumphant return? It's a great story. The transformation was largely the result of one thing: his discovery of, and devotion to, the principles of the Bhagavad Gita. Gandhi himself would later emphasize: It was not just that he *knew* the Gita, but that he actively put its precepts to work in his life. Gandhi studied the Gita constantly. He chanted it, he memorized it, and he practiced its instructions; he took a frayed copy with him everywhere. It became, as he later said, his "spiritual reference book." Everyone who knew him saw this: His longtime secretary, Mahadev Desai, would say, "Every moment of Gandhi's life is a conscious effort to live the message of the Gita."

We might say that M. K. Gandhi engaged in *deliberate practice* of the Bhagavad Gita. He mastered it in just the way that Corot mastered landscape painting, or that Beethoven mastered the sonata form. The battlefield of life described in the opening chapter of the Gita was Gandhi's canvas, and the conversation between Krishna and Arjuna was his instruction book. Gandhi's life, then, must be for us an extraordinary living textbook of the Gita. It is where we will fittingly end our exploration.

— 3 —

Mohandas Gandhi was a fear-obsessed little boy with big eyes, and mammoth ears that stood out almost at right angles from his body. He was terrified of the dark, and, as he said, "haunted by the fear of thieves, ghosts, and serpents." He could not bear to be in a room alone, and could not sleep at night without a light on nearby. Gandhi, later in life, acknowledged that as a boy he had been, in his own words, a "coward." All the other boys on the playground knew it: He was a pushover. One could steal this guy's lunch money with impunity.

And yet, the later Gandhi was fearless. He was renowned not only for his great moral courage, but for physical courage as well. A central pillar of his later teaching was that fearlessness is a prerequisite for nonviolence. "Nonviolence and cowardice go ill together," he said. It is fascinating, then, to dig down into the story of Gandhi's mastery of his fear. How did he accomplish it?

Gandhi himself often told the story. It turns out that as a boy, he was under the care of an old family servant named Rambha. Rambha was touched—and somewhat irritated—by this scrawny kid who came running to her in tears every day after school, pummeled once again by the bullies. She was going to put an end to this.

"It's perfectly all right to admit that you're afraid," she said. "There's no shame in fear. But try this: Whenever you're threatened, instead of running away, stand firm, and repeat the mantra, *Rama, Rama, Rama.* This will turn your fear into courage." *Rama,* of course, is one of the many names of God in the Hindu tradition—and so both the word itself, as well as the *process* of its repetition, had magic in it.

Gandhi-the-boy tried the technique halfheartedly. He found it useful. But he did not discover its true genius until a decade later when Gandhi-the-man was beginning his work with nonviolent noncooperation in South Africa. In the stress of those years he remembered Rambha's advice, and put it to work in earnest. He began to practice the mantra, chanting *Rama, Rama, Rama* over and over again to himself—both aloud and silently. The mantra eased his fear—calmed his mind and body. He began to rely on it, and eventually began to systematically practice chanting mantra not just *in extremis,* but as a part of his regular daily schedule.

For a period of time after this discovery, Gandhi walked many miles each day, repeating the mantra to himself until it began to coordinate itself with the movement of his body and breath. The practice not only calmed him, but brought him into periods of bliss and rapture—and, as he said, "opened the doorway to God." *Rama, Rama, Rama.* Eventually, the mantra developed a life of its own within him. The mantra began to chant itself, arising spontaneously whenever he needed it. "The mantra becomes one's staff of life," he wrote, "and carries one through every ordeal . . . Each repetition . . . has a new meaning, each repetition carries you nearer and nearer to God."

How important was mantra to Gandhi's transformation? Extremely. When done systematically, mantra has a powerful effect on the brain. It gathers and focuses the energy of the mind. It teaches the mind to focus on one point, and it cultivates a steadiness that over time becomes an unshakable evenness of temper. The cultivation of this quality of "evenness" is a central principle of the Bhagavad Gita. It is called *samatva* in Sanskrit, and it is a central pillar of Krishna's practice. When the mind develops steadiness, teaches Krishna, it is not shaken by fear or greed.

So, in his early twenties, Gandhi had already begun to develop a still-point at the center of his consciousness—a still-point that could not be shaken. This little seed of inner stillness would grow into a mighty oak. Gandhi would become an immovable object.

Rambha had given Gandhi an enchanting image to describe the power of mantra. She compared the practice of mantra to the training of an elephant. "As the elephant walks through the market," taught Rambha, "he swings his trunk from side to side and creates havoc with it wherever he goes—knocking over fruit stands and scattering vendors, snatching bananas and coconuts wherever possible. His trunk is naturally restless, hungry, scattered, undisciplined. This is just like the mind—constantly causing trouble."

"But the wise elephant trainer," said Rambha, "will give the elephant a stick of bamboo to hold in his trunk. The elephant likes this. He holds it fast. And as soon as the elephant wraps his trunk around the bamboo, the trunk begins to settle. Now the elephant strides through the market like a prince: calm, collected, focused, serene. Bananas and coconuts no longer distract."

So too with the mind. As soon as the mind grabs hold of the mantra, it begins to settle. The mind holds the mantra gently, and it becomes focused, calm, centered. Gradually this mind becomes extremely concentrated. This is the beginning stage of meditation. All meditation traditions prescribe some beginning practice of gathering, focusing, and concentration—and in the yoga tradition this is most often achieved precisely through mantra.

The whole of Chapter Six in the Bhagavad Gita is devoted to Krishna's teachings on this practice: "Whenever the mind wanders, restless and diffuse in its search for satisfaction without, *lead it within; train it to rest in the Self*," instructs Krishna. "When meditation is mastered, the mind is unwavering like the flame of a lamp in a windless place."

In the midst of Krishna's teaching on meditation, Arjuna whines: "This is too hard! Krishna," he gripes, "the mind is restless, turbulent, powerful, violent; trying to control it is like trying to tame the wind."

Krishna takes a deep breath: "Just keep practicing," he says, and he prescribes "regular practice and detachment."

After Krishna has taught Arjuna the basics of meditation, he makes an important connection for him—a connection that Gandhi will later make as well. When the mind is still, says Krishna, the True Self begins to reveal its nature. In the depths of meditation, we begin to recognize again that we are One with Brahman—that we are that wave that is non-separate from the sea. *Memory is restored!*

In his early twenties, then, Gandhi had already appropriated the meditative tool that would serve him for the rest of his life. He was practicing the only meditation technique taught in the Bhagavad Gita, and was building the foundation of his contemplative practice. In the midst of terrifying circumstances to come, Gandhi held on to the mantra like an elephant grasping bamboo. Friends who knew him well acknowledged that Gandhi repeated his mantra continually, night and day. The name of God invaded the deepest parts of his mind.

—— 4 ——

Gandhi graduated from high school with an underwhelming record, and he went on to college, falteringly. There, too, he failed. After five months he gave up, dropped out, and came home. Gandhi's family was worried: This boy was on the brink of becoming a serious loser—more of a ne'er-do-well than even Thoreau. (No credit to his town!) As a last resort, an uncle suggested that Gandhi go to London to study the law.

What could go wrong with this plan? Plenty. Gandhi fared no better in London. He felt out of place. His textbook English did not suffice. He was more socially inept than ever. For a while he tried to masquerade as an English gentleman. This ruse, however, was patently laughable. He looked ridiculous in his high starched collars, with his enormous ears protruding just above.

In London, Gandhi suffered a painful identity crisis. Who the heck was he? Who was he meant to be in this world? During this period, a desperate Gandhi launched himself into an intense investigation of world religions—searching for answers. He was acutely aware that his life had no unifying principle. Like Arjuna, *he did not understand how to act.* He read the Bible, but was bored with everything except the Sermon on the Mount (which, he said, overwhelmed him with its obvious truth). He looked into Theosophy. He read parts of the Koran. He attended various spiritual groups. But it was not until a young English friend introduced him to the Bhagavad Gita that he felt he had connected with something important. He would never forget his first reading of the Gita. "It went straight to my heart," he declared.

Why, he wondered, had he not read it before? To his shame, he later said, he had not read "Mother Gita" in India, but had to come to London to read it with English friends, in an English translation. "What effect this reading of the Gita had on my friends, only they can say," he wrote, "but to me the Gita became an infallible guide of conduct. It became my dictionary of daily reference. Just as I turned to the English dictionary for the meanings of English words that I did not understand, I turned to this dictionary of conduct for a ready solution of all my troubles and trials."

Gandhi, of course, identified with Arjuna. He was often overcome by doubt, and perpetually on the floor of his own chariot. But he found that reading Mother Gita took some of the rough edges off his self-division. It unified him. "When doubts haunt me, when disappointments stare me in the face, and I see not one ray of hope, I turn to the Bhagavad Gita, and find a verse to comfort me; and I begin to smile in the midst of overwhelming sorrow."

Is it a coincidence that Mohandas Gandhi's life force began to stir at precisely the time he discovered the Gita? I don't think so. The scripture startled him. It woke him up.

By his midtwenties, two of the pillars of Gandhi's transformation were in place: his mantra and his spiritual reference book. With these two, Gandhi began to throw off what he later called the "sluggishness" and "drowsiness" of his mind and body. He would soon discover the third pillar of his transformation: the systematic cultivation of energy.

— 5 —

As he woke up, Gandhi became interested in ways to build strength and resilience in his eighty-pound-weakling body. Gandhi, very much like

Thoreau before him, began to create what he called "experiments in living." His first series of experiments centered around diet. In London, he fell in with a group of vegetarians, and he became fascinated with the health-giving effects of "eating no living beings." He tried every conceivable combination of fruits and vegetables, of beans and rice. What food would give him the most energy, the most stamina? He gave up eating as a recreation and took it up as a spiritual practice. No more living to eat. Now, it was eating to live.

Gandhi found that he felt most energetic when he ate sparsely. Eventually he would settle on goat's milk and vegetables as the diet that gave him the most vitality. (His diet became notorious in India. When, later in life, he was routinely jailed by the viceroy of India, the viceroy himself made sure that the imprisoned Gandhi was always provided with a goat to milk.)

Gandhi was an inveterate experimenter, and he would tinker with his diet for the rest of his life. There are countless stories of friends who came to dine and were given some inedible mélange, which Gandhi at that time believed to be supremely health giving. There was apparently much rolling of eyes at these dinners. Gandhi was not interested in taste, but in effect. He discovered, he said, an "inner relish, distinctly more healthy, delicate, and permanent than food."

In London, Gandhi began, too, an experiment in simplifying his life—another way of sustaining his energy. Gandhi had a vegetarian friend—a real minimalist—who lived in one room and cooked his own meals. This was a practice that was unheard of among the scholar class in England. But Gandhi was attracted to the simplicity of this approach. He decided to adopt it himself.

Gandhi rented a single room that was centrally located in London so that he could walk wherever he went, obviating the need for bus fare, and giving him lots of daily exercise. As a result, he walked miles and miles in London, even in the harsh winters. He began to develop the habit of vigorous walking that would last the rest of his life. In this, too, he was like Thoreau, except that Thoreau, famously, "rambled." Gandhi decidedly did not ramble. He practically flew. All of his walking companions commented on this. Gandhi was famous, later in life, for outwalking even his young companions. "His feet barely touched the ground," they would complain. One can only imagine the sight of this somewhat strange-looking little Indian man walking furiously around London, chanting his Sanskrit mantra all the while. Proper London must have been amused.

Gandhi was discovering the power of simplification and renunciation. He stumbled onto a truth widely known by yogis: Every time we discerningly renounce a possession, we free up energy that can be channeled into the pursuit of dharma. Renunciation was never meant to be for its own sake, but for the sake of dharma. Thoreau discovered precisely this same principle at Walden, where he gradually pared away every possession that was not absolutely necessary (Keep only one spoon! Plant fewer beans!) and where he experienced the same resulting increase in energy that Gandhi did.

Gandhi, without knowing it, was beginning to adopt the worldview of the yogi. The yogi's chief concern is with the art of living, systematically cultivating energy and health. More than anything, he is concerned with living an optimal human life. This was becoming Gandhi's concern, too. But for the yogi, this concern comes with a proviso: Optimal health and well being are not for their own sake, but rather to be used in the service of others. This would be Gandhi's next discovery.

— 6 —

Now comes what we might call the end of the beginning of Gandhi's transformation: his fourteen years in South Africa. It was in South Africa that he would discover the fourth leg of the four-legged dharma stool of his life: the ideal of selfless service.

After three years of legal studies in London, Gandhi passed the notoriously easy bar exams, and enrolled in the High Court. He returned to India briefly—just long enough to embarrass himself and his family one more time. He soon left India again, this time for a legal post that had been arranged for him far off in South Africa by another generous uncle.

Early on in his tenure in South Africa, Gandhi stumbled his way into a particularly complex legal case. The case was almost certainly beyond his slim legal skills. However, knowing that if he failed here he might in fact never get another case in South Africa (and thus become a briefless barrister on two continents), he brought every bit of resolve he had to the task. He mastered the complex arguments involved. Some of his London discipline began to pay off.

For the very first time, in his conduct of this case, we see a spark of the later great man. Gandhi found himself defending a client whose argument was strong. But Gandhi knew enough about the law to know that, strong as the argument was, this complex case was likely to drag out for years in the courts, draining the clients while enriching the lawyers. Gandhi had an idea: He implored his client to submit the case to arbitration and to settle out of court (even though Gandhi himself had much to gain financially by continuing the court battle). Gandhi's client and the opposing client were related to each other, and Gandhi could see that with every month that passed, this divided family plunged deeper and deeper into suffering. This moved Gandhi's heart—and his conscience. After much cajoling, Gandhi finally convinced both sides to enter into arbitration. The result was a peaceful ending to the family strife.

Gandhi was ecstatic. "I had learnt," he said, "the true practice of law. I had learnt to find out the better side of human nature and to enter men's hearts. I realized that the true function of a lawyer was to unite parties riven asunder."

To unite parties riven asunder! Gandhi had had the first taste of his dharma. His calling would be to heal separation wherever he found it— separation between family members, between members of different races, between conflicting parties of all kinds. Once he got a taste of this dharma, he was on fire. This is what he could do with his life! For the first time he had a taste of real purpose.

Eknath Easwaran describes the outcome of this discovery: "Without realizing it, Gandhi had found the secret of success. He began to look on every difficulty as an opportunity for service, a challenge that could draw out of him greater resources of intelligence and imagination. In turning his back on personal profit or prestige in his work, he found he had won the trust and even the love of white and Indian South Africans alike."

Gandhi had now encountered the ideal of selfless service. He was seriously lit up. What's more, this work of healing human division and conflict lined up perfectly with the wisdom of the Gita. Now he began to see separation and conflict everywhere, particularly in the suffering of the Indian community in South Africa. He began to identify with the suffering of his community. He devoted more and more of his time to service. The natural culmination of this effort would be his discovery of the principles of *satyagraha,* and his use of mass civil disobedience.

But there was more. His first successful legal case helped him toward another insight. He saw that his energies and intelligence and training did not belong to him. They belonged to the world. He came to believe that a human being is really just a trustee of all that he has—that his gifts are entrusted to him for the good of the world. "My study of English law came to my help," he said. "I understood the Gita teaching of nonpossession to mean that those who desired salvation should act like the trustee who, though having control over great possessions, regards not an iota of them as his own." He saw that true living was *living for the sake of others.* He was freed from the bondage of his awkward, inept, fearful self.

Gandhi grasped the paradox: The more he gave away, the more he had. "He who devotes himself to service with a clear conscience, will day by day grasp the necessity for it in greater measure, and will continually grow richer in faith . . . If we cultivate the habit of doing this service deliberately, our desire for service will steadily grow stronger, and will make not only for our own happiness but that of the world at large."

Out of Gandhi's fantastic discovery of selfless service very quickly emerged many other changes in his life. Gandhi's experiments in truth, and in simple living, now became supercharged. He became fascinated with the results of simplification: The more he gave up, the freer he felt, the more energy he had, and the happier he was. The simpler he got, the simpler he wanted to be.

During this period, Gandhi says about the true *satyagrahi:* "He will take only what he strictly needs and leave the rest. One must not possess anything which one does not really need. It would be a breach of this principle to possess unnecessary foodstuffs, clothing, or furniture. For instance, one must not keep a chair if one can do without it. In observing this principle one is led to a progressive simplification of one's own life."

At first glance, this exaggerated simplification looks like some strange new form of Puritanism. But it wasn't. Gandhi was not doing this as a "should." For Gandhi, it was a direct road to freedom.

⸺ 7 ⸺

At about the time of her retirement from the deanship, our friend Katherine had entered into her own search for truth, not unlike the search Gandhi conducted in London. I suggested that she read Gandhi's autobiography, which she did—and she gradually caught fire with Gandhi's thinking. Katherine particularly identified with Gandhi's discovery of the truth of trusteeship. "You know how one little idea can change your life?" she said to me one day. This one had changed hers.

Katherine had been—indeed still was—a trustee for a number of schools and community institutions. This was a role she played well. She understood what it meant to be responsible for the best use of an organization's assets. In fact, she'd been notoriously ferocious in conserving the assets of every organization on whose board she'd sat. And she understood that the assets were to be used for one thing only: *to maximize the mission.* When she transferred this frame of thinking to her own life, it was as if a light switched on in her brain. She saw that she was the sole trustee of her own gifts, opportunities, and assets. It was up to her to put these to work in the very best interests of the world. What was *her* mission?

I reminded Katherine of Teilhard de Chardin's identical conclusion: "My life does not belong to me." Chardin would have said, "My life belongs to God." Katherine found it closer to the truth to say, "My life belongs to the world." This reframed the struggle of her life. It set her free. As she internalized this insight, she realized that she had made a small but crucial error in her understanding of her life. Up until this point, she had been dedicating her gifts, her assets, and her opportunities, to *herself.* She had taken her *self* as her primary project in life. And this had caused suffering.

One evening she called me, excited. "Stephen, I've discovered something that's probably totally obvious to you." She went on to explain her insight. If you don't find your work in the world and throw yourself wholeheartedly into it, you will *inevitably make your self your work.* There's no way around it: You will take your self as your primary project. You will, in the very best case, dedicate your life to the *perfection* of your self. To the perfection of your health, intelligence, beauty, home, or even spiritual prowess. And the problem is simply this: This self-dedication is too small a work. It inevitably becomes a prison.

Katherine had been startled by this discovery, and she began to see its manifestations everywhere. She saw it, most of all, among her friends. "We're all constantly preoccupied with 'How am I doing?' 'How am I measuring up?'" she said to me. And she realized that no matter how well-perfected it was, her *self* was never going to be enough. She would forever have to struggle with her aging body, her aging mind, and the increasingly limited accomplishments of her day-to-day life. *She* would never be enough!

This insight is brilliantly expressed in the *Tao te Ching*. "Hope and fear," it teaches, "are both phantoms that arise from thinking of the self. When we don't see the self as self, what do we have to fear?"

Then, the author of the *Tao te Ching*, Lao-Tzu, makes a stunning prescription for living a fulfilled life:

See the world as your self.
Have faith in the way things are.
Love the world as your self;
Then you can care for all things.

See the world as your self. Then you can care for all things! As we age, we will always be losing the "How am I doing?" game—the "How am I measuring up?" game. Old age, illness, and death heighten our awareness of the inevitable failure of the self project. It is all going down to the grave. But when we throw ourselves into our work for the world, the project of self—with all its disappointments—disappears. When we lavish our love on the world, it doesn't matter whether we succeed or fail. It's inherently fulfilling.

This was precisely Gandhi's discovery in South Africa. And the insight changed his life. Prior to this, Gandhi had been taking himself as his own project. And he had been a dramatic failure. When he took the world as his project, and gave up any clinging to outcome, he saw that he could not possibly lose.

See the world as your self. Love the world as your self. This is a simple reframe—like taking one small step to the side. You only have to love what you already love. For Katherine: Gardening. Editing. Writing. The magazine. You only have to love your little corner of the world. But you have to do it intentionally. And full out. And you have to get yourself out of the way. *Then you can care for all things.*

Gandhi came to believe that any power he might have to affect the world only emerged when he got himself out of the way, and let God do the work. He came to call this "reducing yourself to zero." "There comes a time," he wrote in the peak of his maturity, "when an individual becomes irresistible and his action becomes all-pervasive in its effects. This comes when he reduces himself to zero."

It's a wonderful phrase. Gandhi's meaning was simple: Only the human being who acts in a way that is *empty of self* can be the instrument of Soul Force. And it is only Soul Force that can establish a harmonious world. Human beings alone are helpless to resolve conflicts without it. With it, however, Gandhi came to believe that harmony is inevitable. Because harmony, Oneness with all beings, is our true nature.

Gandhi discovered to his delight that when his own self was not in the way—when he was not clinging to any fixed views about the outcome of his actions—he could be hugely creative. He was free to move on a dime, very much as Harriet Tubman moved. Like Tubman, Gandhi began to listen carefully to his inner guidance and to trust this guidance. As a result, his actions were highly creative, and also wildly unpredictable. Gandhi himself often had no idea what creative solutions would emerge from his inner guidance—or *when* they would emerge. (In later years, when he was back in India leading the resistance to British domination, he would have all of India waiting with bated breath—sometimes for weeks or months—while he sat quietly in his ashram spinning cotton, praying, and waiting for guidance about the next action.)

Eknath Easwaran wrote about this phenomenon: "Gandhi was the most bewildering opponent any nation ever faced. Every move he made was spontaneous; every year that passed found him more youthful, more radical, more experimental. British administrators were baffled and exasperated by this little man who withdrew when they would have attacked, attacked when they would have withdrawn, and seemed to be getting stronger day by day. No one knew what he was going to do next, for his actions were prompted not by calculations of what seemed politically expedient, but by a deep intuition which often came to him only at the eleventh hour."

— 8 —

Take yourself to zero. Not for yourself, but for the world. Having taken yourself to zero, you are free to act. And Gandhi was a man of action. Indeed, for him, it was *action aligned with truth* that had true power, true Soul Force.

Gandhi identified with Thoreau's near-mystic view of the power of action aligned with Truth. Thoreau, he believed, had fully grasped and articulated his own view of Soul Force. Soul Force means holding to Truth no matter how fierce the storm. Because he wants nothing for himself, the true *satyagrahi* is not afraid of entering any conflict for the sake of those around him—and he enters it without hostility, without resentment, without resorting even to violent words. In the face of the fiercest provocation, he never lets himself forget that he and his attacker are one. This is the true spirit of *ahimsa,* or "nonviolence." But *ahimsa* is more than just the absence of violence: It is the presence of justice and of love. Gandhi always made it perfectly clear that "the *satyagrahi's* object is to convert, not to coerce, the wrongdoer."

In South Africa, Gandhi had brought this understanding to maturity. His movement of nonviolent resistance in South Africa was spectacularly successful. Six years after his first civil disobedience—and after many other such actions—he and the South African president, General Jan Smuts, signed a pact that led, at last, to the so-called "Indian Relief Bill," which restored Indians' civil rights. Gandhi would call it the Magna Carta of South African Indians, and it was a mammoth victory for Soul Force.

— 9 —

By the year 1915 Gandhi knew that he was complete with his work in South Africa. He felt called to return to India, where his people were suffering under the increasingly onerous burden of British rule. Gandhi returned to India a seasoned veteran of *satyagraha,* and he believed that the principles he had tried so successfully in South Africa could be put into action in India. He believed that they would inevitably result in the political freedom and self-determination of the Indian people. He knew that this could be done without war, without violence, and without contempt for the British. And he knew that it was his dharma to lead the way.

Gandhi had left India a fearful, befuddled young attorney. He returned a masterful *satyagrahi.* More than anything else, he had mastered his disabling fear. He had become an exemplar of courage. And he knew that this kind of courage would be required of the whole Indian people in order to throw off British rule. "Greater courage is required of the *satyagrahi,*" he often said, "than the run-of-the mill soldier with a gun in his hand. Any coward can be brave when holding a rifle."

Gandhi's courage surprised no one more than himself. He sometimes wondered just how far his own courage would hold. He really did not know. He wrote: "Have I that nonviolence of the brave in me? My death alone will show that. If someone killed me and I died with a prayer for the assassin on my lips, and God's remembrance and consciousness of His living presence in the sanctuary of my heart, then alone would I be said to have had the nonviolence of the brave."

Krishna taught Arjuna that the origin of all fearlessness is the facing of death. Indeed, their entire conversation took place just on the edge of death—on the edge of the great battlefield on which Arjuna might well die. Gandhi himself had to wrestle with death almost constantly throughout his career. Indeed, it is likely that Gandhi knew he would face a violent death. He wrote presciently: "Death is the appointed end of all life. To die by the hand of a brother rather than by disease or in such other way, cannot be for me a matter of sorrow. And if, even in such a case, I am free from the thought of anger or hatred against my assailant, I know that it will redound to my eternal welfare, and even the assailant will later on realize my perfect innocence."

This is exactly how Gandhi did die, of course. Then seventy-eight years old, he was in Delhi, working—as ever—for unity. He had had a particularly busy day. And as he was hurrying to evening prayers, arm in arm with two young disciples, a young man approached him, offered him a gesture of respect, and then fired a gun point-blank into his heart.

As the Great Soul crumpled to the ground, his mantra emerged spontaneously from his lips: *Rama, Rama, Rama.*

—— 10 ——

For Mahatma Gandhi, all of his courage, all of his trust in God, all of his capacity to love the world as himself issued from the pages of the Bhagavad Gita.

No human being living in the twentieth century has lived the precepts of this great text with more fidelity and passion than Gandhi. "Select your purpose," he challenged, "selfless, without any thought of personal pleasure or personal profit, and then use selfless means to attain your goal."

"Do not resort to violence," Gandhi wrote, "even if it seems at first to promise success; it can only contradict your purpose. Use the means of love and respect even if the result seems far off or uncertain. Then throw yourself heart and soul into the campaign, counting no price too high for working for the welfare of those around you, and every reverse, every defeat, will send you deeper into your own deepest resources. Violence can never bring an end to violence; all it can do is provoke more violence. But if we can adhere to complete nonviolence in thought, word, and deed, India's freedom is assured."

And assured, indeed, it was, largely as a result of the faith and integrity of this one small man who took himself to zero—and who simply put into practice the words of his divine mentor, Krishna.

—— 11 ——

When Gandhi first discovered his dharma—"to unite parties riven asunder"—he realized that this calling would somehow save him—give him something to live for—give him a focus for his life. Gandhi's sacred calling showed up just in the nick of time. It appeared to him as a lifeboat in a stormy sea. At last! Something reliable to cling to. Something that actually floats. Beethoven's music occurred for him, too, as a welcome raft in a gale. And Keats's poetry. And Mark's playwriting.

Many of us have precisely this experience of dharma: a lifeboat! You cling to it because it is the only boat you have and the storm is rising. You work at it—you row as hard as you possibly can against the storm, because you have to survive. But gradually the seas calm, and you don't have to row quite so hard, and you actually begin to enjoy the exercise. You get stronger from the exertion—as Gandhi did. Finally, the storm abates. You have a spell of beautiful weather. You feel your strength. You begin to love this rowing. You begin to love the sea itself. You see things in the waves that others do not see. You begin to see that rowing this little boat of dharma connects you to very life. Gradually the task of rowing itself begins to ease. At times it is effortless. There are moments of rapture.

Dharma is very much like Gandhi's mantra. *Rama, Rama, Rama.* Eventually it takes on a life of its own. It does things spontaneously that you had no reason to expect. It begins to drill down into the deepest parts of your mind. Soon you begin to see that this dharma is not just any old stick of bamboo. It is a magic wand. A wish-fulfilling wand. It is a way to *know*—to interact with, to be in relationship with—the deepest parts of yourself. It is a vehicle to know the world.

Eventually your dharma takes you into a new land, as Gandhi's did. A land where you can rely only upon God. You cross a bridge, and you are suspended in the air. Only God is holding you up now.

"Abandon all supports," says Krishna to Arjuna in one of his great final teachings. "Cast off your dependency on everything external, Arjuna, and rely on the Self alone."

We work first because we have to work. Then because we want to work. Then because we love to work. Then the work simply does us. Difficult at the beginning. Inevitable at the end.

—— EPILOGUE ——

Krishna and Arjuna have now reached the end of their dialogue. It's twilight on the battlefield of Kurukshetra. There's a cool breeze moving over the now-quiet field, bringing a faint smell of the river that lies beyond. Arjuna has gotten up to stretch, and to bring a cup of water to Krishna, who is seated under a small banyan tree at the edge of the field.

As Arjuna sits down on a log next to Krishna, they both realize that the wondrous dialogue has reached its conclusion. How long have they sat here talking? For weeks? For months? For years? Arjuna really does not know. It seems as though lifetimes have elapsed.

Krishna turns his head to look directly into Arjuna's eyes, and asks, "Have you understood the teaching? Have you listened with attention? Are you now free from your doubts and confusion?"

Arjuna hardly knows how to answer. The whole dialogue seems like an intense and vivid dream. Arjuna knows, though, that he has been mysteriously transformed. "My memory has been restored!" he cries. Through communing with Krishna, *he has remembered who he really is.* Arjuna is no longer deluded into thinking that he is his mortal body, or his personality, or even his various tasks and roles, noble as they are. He knows that his True Self is unborn, is undying, uncreated—immortal.

But the most important outcome is this: Having remembered who he is, Arjuna now knows how to act. Remember that from its very opening sentences, the Bhagavad Gita has been a treatise on action. *When you know who you are, you will know how to act.*

Arjuna returns Krishna's gaze with a faint smile. He feels a wave of gratitude wash through him. "You have dispelled my doubts and delusions," he says, "and I understand through your grace. My faith is firm now, and I will do your will." Arjuna is no longer paralyzed by doubt. He is ready to move back into action. But it will now be action with a difference: It will be action guided by the voice of the Inner Divine.

Krishna, in the final chapter of the Gita, describes the magnificently transformed Arjuna: "Free from self-will, aggressiveness, arrogance, anger, and the lust to possess people or things, he is at peace with himself and others and enters into the unitive state. United with Brahman, ever joyful, beyond the reach of desire and sorrow, he has equal regard for every living creature and attains supreme devotion to me. By loving me he comes to know me truly; then he knows my glory and enters into my boundless being. All his acts are performed in my service, and through my grace he wins eternal life."

— 2 —

Arjuna looks again at the field of Kurukshetra. He anticipates the massing armies that will come with the morning. He perceives again the odor of war.

You have been wondering how the story ends. Will Arjuna fight the battle?

Arjuna will fight, yes. But what is the real nature of this fight? At the outset of our tale, Arjuna saw at Kurukshetra only the great battlefield of a conventional war. Now he has new eyes. He sees that the battle Krishna has called him to fight is really the battle of life. And this battle is revealed to be the *battle of separation*—the separation of sons from fathers, the separation of cousins from uncles, the separation of caste, the separation of race. But most of all, the separation from God.

Arjuna is still a warrior. But his duty now is to fight a different kind of battle. Henceforth he will be engaged with all of his might and passion and skillfulness in the moral equivalent of war.

—— 3 ——

So, we have reached the end of our journey together. Of course, the Bhagavad Gita is just a tale. But do its teachings bear out in real life? In your life?

If you bring forth what is within you it will save you.

Do you think this is so?

My own view is this: There are some things, alas, from which we cannot be saved. Indeed, we cannot be saved from *most* of the things from which we most desperately *want* to be saved. We cannot really be saved from pain, from loss, from failure, from dissatisfaction. We cannot be saved from grasping and aversion.

And yet, dharma clearly *does* save us in many wonderful ways. Dharma saves us not by ending but rather by *redeeming* our suffering. It gives meaning to our suffering. It enables us to bear our suffering. And, most important, it enables our suffering to bear fruit for the world.

I have come to believe that dharma gives us the one thing we need to be fully human: Each of us must have one domain, one small place on the globe where we can fully meet life—where we can meet it with every gift we have. One small place where, through testing ourselves, we can *know* the nature of life, and ultimately know ourselves. This domain, this one place that is uniquely ours, is our *work in the world.* Our work in the world is for each of us the *axis mundi,* the immovable spot—the one place where we really have the opportunity to wake up.

Dharma provides us with the perfect vehicle through which we can fruitfully die to our smaller self and be reborn to Self. And make no mistake: This mystic death—this death that our egos abhor—this taking ourselves to zero—is absolutely required in order to be fully human.

My good friend Luke is a Christian monk, living in a monastery not too far from Kripalu. He tells me that the most important work of his life—his work of prayer, his dharma—mostly takes place in his little ten-by-ten monk's room. In his tradition, this little room is called a "cell." Luke also sometimes refers to his little cell as his "tomb." For a while I thought he was joking about this. But no. In his tradition the monks are told early on: "Your cell is your tomb where you die and arise to new life."

Luke showed me his cell one day. It was simple, sparsely furnished, whitewashed. But that simplicity belied the complex work that I knew went on there. Prayer is hard work. I could practically see the gnash marks in the white plaster walls. As you pit yourself against any real dharma, the problems of mastery, the challenges of selflessness, and the need for sustained courage all arise. In every case, the authentic pursuit of dharma results in gnash marks. Your dharma is your tomb where you die and arise to new life. You only *get* yourself when you lose yourself to some great work. And whatever your authentic work is—I believe it *is* great. It is the great work of your life.

—— 4 ——

Do you have a sense that you know more about your dharma now than when we began this journey together, twelve chapters ago? I hope so.

As for me, I can say that studying the lives of Goodall and Thoreau, of Lonny and Ethan and Mark, of Corot and Tubman and Gandhi, has helped me tremendously. It has helped me resolve my midlife confusion about dharma—the confusion I spoke about in the Introduction to this book. I see now that I had been confused about dharma because I had both too *high* an opinion of it and too *low* an opinion of it all at the same time. I thought that life should always be high art. I thought, indeed, that I should always be jumping out of bed in the morning, ripping open the curtain to meet the day. When we study the lives of truly fulfilled exemplars of dharma, we discover that, alas, it is just not like that, even for the most accomplished among them.

I have come to see that dharma is more like craft than high art. Those of us struggling to live our dharmas awake every morning like everyone else—to the sound of the alarm. We roll over. We take a deep breath. Another day. We know what we have to do. We get up. We make the coffee. We work away at the work we were put here and set here to do, like plodding, persistent craftsmen—putting one foot in front of the other. We are part of a team of craftsmen building a cathedral. We may not live to see the whole structure completed. In fact, our small part of the magnificent whole may not even be visible to the eye once the thing is finished. No matter. It is not really about us anyway. It is about the cathedral.

Through studying the many extraordinary lives that appear in these pages, I have come to see that our understanding of dharma today is obscured by our fondness for the cult of personality and for self and for celebrity. Our understanding of dharma is obscured by the narcissism of our time. Studying the lives of great exemplars of dharma has helped me to see that the primary distortion in my dharma life has been the age-old misery of self-absorption. Deep in midlife I had begun to feel the awful burden of wanting to be special; wanting to be better; wanting to experience every possible adventure in this life; wanting to be, as we have sometimes said at Kripalu, an "expanded self."

Oh, for God's sake. It is just too damned much work to be an expanded self. Couldn't I just be an ordinary self?

The great twentieth-century monk Thomas Merton encountered precisely the same spiritual exhaustion partway through his life. The chief source of this exhaustion, he writes, "is the selfish anxiety to get the most out of everything, to be a sparkling success in our own eyes and in the eyes of other men." His vision of the possibility of relief from this burden occurred to me as brilliant: "We can only get rid of this anxiety by being content to miss something in almost everything we do."

What? Miss something in almost everything we do? That is allowed?

Merton says it is: "We cannot master everything, taste everything, understand everything, drain every experience to its last dregs. But if we have the courage to let almost everything else go, we will probably be able to retain the one thing necessary for us—whatever it may be. If we are too eager to have everything, we will almost certainly miss even the one thing we need."

This has the feel of truth to me. A difficult truth. But a truth that may free me from the obviously false hope that I *can* have everything—indeed, from the view that I *must* have everything in order to have a fulfilling life.

Authentic dharma frees us from this false hope. Merton sees deeply into the nature of this freedom: ". . . the fulfillment of every individual vocation demands not only the renunciation of what is evil in itself, but also of all the precise goods that are not willed for us by God." We are not called to *everything*. We are just called to what we're called to. It is inevitable that authentically good parts of ourselves will not be fulfilled. What a relief.

"We can do no great things," wrote the nineteenth-century French saint, Teresa, "only small things with great love."

Thomas Merton—who struggled through his whole life with his longing to be considered a great author—writes of this: ". . . we cannot achieve greatness unless we lose all interest in being great. For our own idea of greatness is illusory, and if we pay too much attention to it we will be lured out of the peace and stability of the being God gave us, and seek to live in a myth we have created for ourselves. It is, therefore, a very great thing to be little, which is to say: to be ourselves. And when we are truly ourselves we lose most of the futile self-consciousness that keeps us constantly comparing ourselves with others in order to see how big we are."

Merton here catches exactly the spirit of Thoreau and Anthony and Tubman—and all the others. These great exemplars of dharma each took a craftsmanlike view toward life: Do your daily duty, and let the rest go. Poke away systematically at your little calling. Tend the garden a little bit every day. You do not have to exhaust yourself with great acts. Show up for your duty, for your dharma. Then let it go.

In monasteries of old, the monk's dharma, his purpose in life, was said to be this: *to support the choir*. In Latin, *propter chorum*. Literally, his life was lived "in support of the choir." He was not a soloist. He was not a diva. He was part of a magnificent whole.

— 5 —

The holy dialogue between Krishna and Arjuna is at an end. It has been so powerful that it has transformed all who have listened to it. Sanjaya himself the narrator of "the wondrous dialogue"—has been changed by it. Just recalling the scene of their dialogue lights him up with ecstasy. "The wonder of it makes my hair stand on end!" he exclaims.

"Whenever I remember these wonderful, holy words between Krishna and Arjuna, I am filled with joy," he says. "And when I remember the breathtaking form of Krishna, I am filled with wonder and my joy overflows."

Sanjaya speaks the final words: "Wherever the divine Krishna and the mighty Arjuna are, there will be prosperity, victory, happiness, and sound judgment. Of this I am sure!"

—— NOTES ——

Epigraph

ix "Every man has a vocation" Thomas Merton. *No Man Is an Island.* Harcourt Brace Jovanovich: New York, 1978, p. 133.

Introduction

xv "What you fear is" Thomas Merton. *A Year with Thomas Merton: Daily Meditations from His Journals,* Thomas Merton, Jonathan Montaldo. HarperCollins: New York, p. 178.

xvi "If you bring forth" "The Gospel of Thomas" 45: 29–33, see Elaine Pagels. *The Gnostic Gospels.* Vintage: New York, 1989, p. xv.

xx "All that is worthwhile" Teilhard de Chardin, quoted in *For the Time Being,* Annie Dillard. Alfred A. Knopf: New York, 1999, p. 105.

PART I: Krishna's Counsel on the Field of Battle

3 "I see omens of chaos" Barbara Stoler Miller. *The Bhagavad Gita: Krishna's Counsel in Time of War.* Bantam: New York, 1986, I.31, p. 25.

4 "Krishna, halt my chariot" ibid., I.21, 22, pp. 23–24.

4 "fathers, grandfathers, teachers" ibid., I.26, p. 24.

5 "Conflicting sacred duties" ibid., 2.7, p. 30.

5 "We don't know which" ibid., 2.6, p. 30.

5 "My limbs sink" ibid., I.29, 30, p. 25.

6 "I cannot fight" Author's translation of, *The Bhagavad Gita,* 2.9.

ONE

8 "Doubt afflicts the person" Author's translation, *Gita*, 4.40.

8 "Doubt is a state in which" Charles B. Herbermann et al, eds. *The Catholic Encyclopedia*. Vol. 5. Robert Appleton Company: New York, 1909, p. 141.

8 "Doubt is opposed to certitude" ibid., p. 141.

9 "Krishna, my delusion is destroyed" Stoler Miller, *Gita*, 18.73, p. 153.

15 "No one exists" ibid., 3.5, p. 41.

15 "OK . . . so I cannot" Occasionally, as in this case, the author has imagined or paraphrased a statement by Arjuna.

15 "Arjuna, look to" Author's translation, *Gita*, 2.31.

15 "There is a certain" The author imagines this speech, based on the text.

16 "Look to your" Stoler Miller, *Gita*, 2.31, p. 34.

16 "Relinquish the fruits" Author's translation, *Gita*, 18.2, p. 143.

16 "It is better" ibid., 3.35, p. 46.

16 "Dedicate your actions" ibid., 3.30, p. 33.

PART II: The First Pillar: "Look to Your Dharma"

21 "Dharma is the essential" René Guénon. *Introduction to the Study of Hindu Doctrines*. Sophia Perennis: Hillsdale, NY, 2001, p. 146.

TWO

29 "The gentlest thing" Stephen Mitchell. *Tao te Ching*. Harper Perennial: New York, 1991, saying 43.

30 "One of my tasks" Jane Goodall. *Reason for Hope: A Spiritual Journey*. Warner Books: New York, 2000, p. 6.

30 "At last, a hen" ibid., p. 6.

31 "despite her worry" ibid., pp. 6–7.

32 "I was lucky" ibid., p. 7.

32 "assumed, upon depositing" paraphrase, based on ibid., p. 61.

32 "Little did they" ibid., p. 61.

32 "I had a mother" ibid., p. 4.

34 "The attempt to live" author's paraphrase.

35 "As David and I sat" Goodall, Hope, p. 81.

36 "More and more" ibid., p. 81.

36 "Each one of us" ibid., p. 266.

36 "Of course, it is" ibid., p. 267.

36 "I always have" ibid., p. 267.

36 "The youth gets together" Henry David Thoreau, from his *Journal*, July 14, 1852.

37 "Play comes after" paraphrased from *Walden*, Chapter I.

THREE

39 "Be resolutely and faithfully" Henry David Thoreau. *Journal,* ed. John C. Broderick et al. Vol. I. Princeton University Press: Princeton, NJ, 1981, p. 225.

39 "Depend upon it" Henry David Thoreau, quoted in Stoler Miller, *Gita,* p. 161.

39 "A man tracks himself" Henry David Thoreau, quoted in Robert T. Richardson, Jr. *Henry Thoreau, A Life of the Mind.* University of California Press: Berkeley, 1986, p. 291.

40 "A man's own calling" Henry David Thoreau, quoting Krishna, in *A Week on the Concord and Merrimack Rivers,* quoted in Stoler Miller, *Gita,* p. 156.

40 "an irresponsible idler" Richardson, *Thoreau,* p. 298.

41 "Thoreau is as ugly" Nathaniel Hawthorne, from *American Notebooks,* September 1, 1842, quoted in *Bloom's Classic Critical Views: Henry David Thoreau.* Bloom's Literary Criticism: New York, 2008, p. 8.

44 "Think of the small as large" Mitchell, *Tao te Ching,* Saying 63.

44 "See yourself as a grain of sand" paraphrased from Chögyam Trungpa Rinpoche, *The Myth of Freedom and the Way of Meditation.* Shambhala: Boston, 1976, p. 9.

45 "human nature in general" Richardson, *Thoreau,* p. 74.

45 "Self-emancipation in the" Thoreau, from his *Journal,* quoted in Richardson, *Thoreau,* p. 152.

46 "The whole is in each man" ibid., *Thoreau,* p. 22.

46 "Imagine this web" Alan Watts, from Alan Watts Podcast: *Following the Middle Way #3,* alanwattspodcast.com

47 "Every object" Sir Charles Eliot, quoted in David Mumford. *Indra's Pearls: The Vision of Felix Klein.* Cambridge University Press: Cambridge, 2002, p. xix.

47 "Dharma upholds" *The Mahabharata,* 12.110.11.

47 "[Thoreau] produced" Richardson, *Thoreau,* p. 154.

48 "I am a mystic" Thoreau, ibid., *Thoreau,* p. 285.

48 "Do what you love!" Thoreau, ibid., p. 188.

50 "If I knew for a certainty" Henry David Thoreau, quoted in Jeffrey S. Cramer. *Walden: A fully annotated edition.* Yale University Press: New Haven, 2004, p. 71.

FOUR

52 The Civil War "saved" This chapter relies heavily throughout on the argument made by Roy Morris, Jr. in his brilliant examination of Whitman's life as a volunteer in the hospitals of the Civil War, presented in his *The Better Angel.* Oxford University Press: Oxford, 2000, p. 3.

52 "Guilty of that horrible" Jerome Loving. *Walt Whitman: The Song of Himself.* University of California Press: Berkeley, 1999, pp. 184–185.

53 "I only gave myself" Whitman, quoted in Morris, *Angel,* p. 5.

53 "launch of a great" Emerson, quoted in Justin Kaplan. *Walt Whitman: A Life.* Simon & Schuster: New York, 1979, p. 203.

53 "I celebrate myself" Walt Whitman in Lawrence Clark Powell. *Poems of Walt Whitman, Leaves of Grass.* Thomas Y. Crowell Company: New York, 1964, p. 72.

54 "I loaf and invite" Whitman in Powell, *Leaves,* p. 72.

56 "I go around from" Walt Whitman, Walter Loenfels, Nan Braymer. *Walt Whitman's Civil War.* DaCapo Press: New York, 1989, p. 101.

57 "his glassy eyes" Whitman, quoted in Morris, *Angel,* p. 86

57 "I sat down by him" Whitman, Loenfels, Braymer, *Whitman,* p. 90.

57 "I cannot give up" Walt Whitman, Edward Haviland Miller, *Selected Letters of Walt Whitman.* University of Iowa Press: Des Moines, 1990, p. 49.

59 "fortifying myself with" Walt Whitman, *Complete Prose Works: Walt Whitman.* [1897] Cornell University Library: Ithaca, 2009, p. 62.

59 "Behold, I do not give" Walt Whitman. *Leaves of Grass.* Sherman and Co: New York, 1881, p. 66.

59 "a silent dark-skinn'd" Whitman, quoted in Morris, *Angel,* p. 127.

59 "Many nights I sat" Walt Whitman, Edward Haviland Miller. *Selected Letters of Walt Whitman.* University of Iowa Press: Des Moines, 1990, p. 78.

59 "I write you this" Walt Whitman, John Harmon McElroy. *The Sacrificial Years: A Chronicle of Walt Whitman's Experiences in the Civil War.* David R. Godine, Publisher, 1999, p. 54.

60 "to express in a poem" Whitman, Haviland, *Whitman,* p. 109.

60 "I see behind each mask" Whitman, *Leaves,* p. 251.

60 "Our bodies are known" Stoler Miller, *Gita,* 2.18, p. 32.

60 "Weapons do not cut" ibid., 2.23, p. 32.

60 "it is enduring" ibid., 2.24, p. 33.

62 "Old men ought to be" T. S. Eliot, *Four Quartets,* in Sunil Kumar Sarker. *T. S. Eliot: Poetry, Plays and Prose.* Atlantic: New Delhi, 1995, 2008, p. 140.

62 "Our bodies are known" Stoler Miller, *Gita,* 2.18, p. 32.

62 "He was assassinated" Whitman, quoted in Morris, *Angel,* p. 221.

63 "Come lovely and" Whitman in Harold Bloom. *Walt Whitman: Bloom's Modern Critical Views.* Chelsea House: New York, 2006, p. 104.

63 "Strive constantly to serve" *The Bhagavad Gita: Translated for the Modern Reader by Eknath Easwaran.* Nilgiri Press: Tomales, California, 1985, 3.19, p. 77.

63 "There were years" David S. Reynolds. *Walt Whitman.* Oxford University Press: USA, 2005, p. 127.

PART III: The Second Pillar: "Do It Full Out!"

67 "From around the age of" Hokusai, quoted in Seiji Nagata. *Hokusai: Genius of the Japanese Ukiyo-e.* Kodansha International: Tokyo, 2000, p. 87.

67 "I became an artist" Hokusai, in Nagata, *Hokusai,* p. 87.

68 "If only heaven" Hokusai, quoted in George Newnes. *The Strand Magazine,* Vol. 15, Jan 1898 No. 85. George Newnes, Ltd: London, 1898, p. 562.

69 "Considering your dharma" Easwaran, *Gita,* 2.31, p. 64.

69 "The ignorant, indecisive" ibid., 4.40, p. 89.

69 "Don't waste time" Guan Yin Tzu, quoted in Timothy Freke. *Taoist Wisdom: Daily Teachings from the Taoist Master.* Sterling: NY, 2002, p. 123.

69 "One of the few things" Annie Dillard. *The Writing Life.* HarperCollins: New York, 1989, p. 78.

70 "The disunited mind" Easwaran, *Gita,* 2.66, p. 68.

70 "must overcome the confusion" ibid., 2.52, p. 67.

FIVE

73 "Two roads diverged" Robert Frost. "The Road Not Taken." *Mountain Interval.* Henry Holt: New York, 1915, p. 9.

74 "For me the initial delight" Frost, quoted in Edward C. Lathem, Lawrence R. Thompson. *The Robert Frost Reader: Poetry and Prose.* Holt Paperback: New York, 2002, p. 440.

74 "meets himself" Frost, in Lathem, *Frost Reader,* p. 440.

74 "Some say the world" Robert Frost. "Fire and Ice," *Harper's Magazine,* December 1920, p. 67.

75 "They would not find me" Robert Frost, in Lawrence Untermeyer. *The Road Not Taken: A Selection of Robert Frost's Poems.* Holt: New York, 2002, p. xxiv.

76 "I liked to try myself" Deirdre J. Fagan. *Critical Companion to Robert Frost.* Facts on File: New York, 2007, p. 5.

76 "Ossian, Poe, Wordsworth, Longfellow, and Bryant" Frost quoted in Jay Parini, *Robert Frost: A Life.* Henry Holt: New York, p. 44.

76 "I wrote it all" Natalie S. Bober. *A Restless Spirit: The Story of Robert Frost.* Henry Holt: New York, 1998, p. 49.

76 "something was happening" ibid., p. 42.

76 "The most demanding" Annie Dillard. *The Writing Life.* HarperCollins: New York, 1989, p. 68.

77 "To love poetry is to" Parini, *Frost,* p. 44.

77 "Specifically speaking, the few" K. Harris. *Robert Frost: Studies of the Poetry.* G. K. Hall and Co., 1980, p. 4.

78 "a more elevated" Parini, *Frost,* p. 45.

79 "Perhaps when that preacher" Peter James Stanlis. *Robert Frost: The Poet as Philosopher.* Second Edition. Intercollegiate Studies Institute, 2008, p. xiii.

79 "talk songs" Parini, *Frost,* p. 76.

79 "is lifted just enough" ibid., p. 77.

79 "sound of sense" ibid., p. 77.

79 "The sound of" Jesse Zuba, Harold Bloom. *Robert Frost: Bloom's Modern Critical Views.* Chelsea House: London, 2003, p. 208.

82 "From all sides" Parini, *Frost,* p. 72.

82 "This was a time" ibid., p. 91.

82 "It was a necessary" ibid., p. 85.

82 "It all started" ibid., p. 72.

84 "No man can know" ibid., p. 115.

85 "a life that followed" ibid., p. 113.

85 "Until one is committed" W. A. Murray. *The Scottish Himalayan Expedition.* J. M. Dent and Sons Ltd: London, 1951, p. 6.

SIX

89 "singleness of purpose" Easwaran, *Gita,* 2.41, p. 65.

89 "For those who lack" ibid., p. 65.

89 "disunited" ibid., 2.66, p. 68.

90 focus as an essential Stephen Covey. *The Seven Habits of Highly Successful People.* Free Press: New York, 1989, p. 9.

90 "winners focus, losers spray" Sydney J. Harris. *Winners and Losers.* Argus Communications: New York, 1973, p. 2.

94 "These old Bachelors" Jean H. Baker. *Sisters: The Lives of America's Suffragists.* Hill and Wang: New York, 2006, p. 62.

94 "When I am crowned" Elizabeth Cady Stanton. *Eighty Years and More: 1815–1898, Reminiscences of Elizabeth Cady Stanton.* Indy Publishing, 2004, p. 172.

94 "I will show you" Charlotte Brontë in Elizabeth Cleghorn Gaskell. *The Life of Charlotte Brontë: Vol II.* Smith, Elder and Co: London, 1857, p. 11.

95 "The true woman will" Susan B. Anthony, in Lynn Sherr. *Failure Is Impossible: Susan B. Anthony in Her Own Words.* Times Books: Toronto, 1995, p. 297.

95 "I am tired of theory" Ann M. Todd. *Susan B. Anthony: Activist.* Chelsea House: London, 2008, p. 27.

96 "the sisters were not" Susan B. Anthony, quoted in Kathleen Barry. *Susan B. Anthony: A Biography of a Singular Feminist.* First Books: Bloomington, IN, 2000, p. 71.

96 "We are heartily sick and tired" Susan B. Anthony, in *Elizabeth Cady Stanton: The Right Is Ours.* Oxford University Press: USA, 2001, p. 61.

97 "Dress loose, take a" ibid., p. 61.

97 "I have no doubt" Susan B. Anthony, Susan Brownell Anthony, Ann D. Gordon. *The Selected Papers of Elizabeth Cady Stanton and Susan B. Anthony, Vol. 4.* Rutgers University Press: Rutgers, 1997, p. 198.

97 "it is most invigorating" Ida Husted Harper. *The Life and Work of Susan B. Anthony, Vol I.* University of Michigan Library: Ann Arbor, 1898, p. 66.

98 "Take a concrete issue" Barry, *Anthony,* p. 76.

98 "With a degree of impiety" Sherr, *Failure,* p. 146.

99 "The mob represents more" Anthony in Barry, *Anthony,* p. 83.

99 "The important thing" ibid., p. 91.

99 "This was the real" ibid.

99 "Susan B. Anthony came to" ibid., p. 111.

100 "[The Master] doesn't glitter" Stephen Mitchell. *Tao te Ching.* HarperPerennial: New York, 1991, Saying 39.

100   "While we differ widely" Geoffrey C. Ward. *Not for Ourselves Alone: The Story of Elizabeth Cady Stanton and Susan B. Anthony—An Illustrated History.* Knopf: New York, 1999.

100   "She did not mince words" Barry, *Anthony,* p. 114.

101   "Until women are made" Anthony in Sherr, *Failure,* p. 66.

101   "Woman and her" ibid., p. 61.

101   "failure is impossible" ibid., xiii.

101   "Not in our day" Anthony in Barry, *Anthony,* p. 132.

102   "Do you pray" Sherr, *Failure,* Chapter 20 "Divine Discontent."

102   Just three years details of scene imagined by the author, drawing on fact, see Barry, *Anthony,* p. xi.

103   "When a person" Easwaran, *Gita,* 7.21, p. 117.

105   "How you spend your" Dillard, *Writing,* p. 32.

SEVEN

107   "so many great works" Monet, quoted in Madeleine Hours. *Jean-Baptiste-Camille Corot.* The Easton Press: Norwalk, CT, 1984, pp. 41-42.

107   "There is only one" ibid., p. 42.

107   "This is the saddest" ibid., p. 42.

107   *In the Light of Italy* This exhibition was held at the National Gallery of Art, Washington, D.C., May 29–September 2, 1996.

107   "They are an idea of an" Robert Frost, quoted in Parini, *Frost,* p. 283.

108   "the artist had captured" Corot, quoted in Patrick Noon. *Crossing the Channel: British and French Painting in the Age of Romanticism.* Tate Publishing: Mustang, OK, 2003, p. 201.

108   "to pursue your" Hours, *Corot,* p. 30.

109   "Do you really think" ibid., p. 30.

109   "Do not follow others" Corot, quoted in Everard Meynell. *Corot and His Friends.* Methuen and Co: London, 1908, p. 97.

112   "You could not imagine" Corot, quoted in Peter Galassi. *Corot in Italy: Open-air Painting and the Classical Landscape Tradition.* Yale University Press: New Haven, 1991, p. 136.

114   "Corot is our master" ibid., p. 152.

114   "One must be severe" ibid.

114   "Many of Corot's best" ibid., p. 191.

117   "Expert Performance" K. Anders Ericsson and Neil Charness. "Expert Performance: Its Structure and Acquisition," *American Psychologist,* Vol. 49, No. 8, August 1994, pp. 725–747.

122   "All I really want" Corot, quoted in Linello Venturi. *Corot: 1796–1875.* Philadelphia Museum of Art: Philadelphia, 1946, p. 20.

122   "Ceaseless work, either" Corot, quoted in Keith Roberts. *Jean-Baptiste-Camille Corot: 1796–1875.* Spring Books: London, 1965, p. 33.

122   "I could be gay" Corot, quoted in Meynell, *Corot,* p. 76.

123   "When you write" Dillard, *Writing,* p. 3.

123   "All must be governed" Corot, quoted in Roberts, *Corot,* p. 37.

123   "You have no idea of the things" Corot, quoted in Meynell, *Corot,* p. 31.

PART IV: The Third Pillar: "Let Go of the Fruits"

127   "You have the right to work" Easwaran, *Gita,* 2.47, p. 66.

127   "You should never engage" ibid., p. 66.

128   "Those who are motivated" ibid., 2.49, p. 66.

129   "When you keep thinking" ibid., 2.62, p. 68.

129   "Seek refuge in the" ibid., 2.49, p. 66.

130   "Neither agitated by" ibid., 2.56, p. 67.

130   "When consciousness is unified" ibid., 2.49, p. 66.

130   "When you move" ibid., 2.62., p. 68.

EIGHT

136   "O, for ten years" John Keats, "Sleep and Poetry," first published 1816. All references to Keats's poems are from H. W. Garrod, Ed. *The Poetical Works of John Keats,* second Oxford edition. Oxford University Press: Oxford, 1958.

136   "The genius of poetry" Keats, in Stuart M. Sperry. *Keats the Poet.* Princeton University Press: Princeton, NJ, 1994, p. 97.

137   "characteristic backward toss" Aileen Ward. *John Keats: The Making of a Poet.* Viking Press: New York, 1967, p. 64.

137   "a particularly dauntless expression" William Sharp. *Life and Letters of Joseph Severn.* University of Michigan Library: Ann Arbor, 1892, p. 20.

138   "He was not one" Ward, *Keats,* p. 44.

139   "Beauty that must die" John Keats, "Ode to Melancholy."

140   "Poetry comes from" Ward, *Keats,* p. 16.

141   "discovered that he had" Geoffrey Treasure, ed. *Who's Who in British History: Beginnings to 1901.* Routledge: London, 1998, p. 748.

142   "the only thing worthy" Walter Jackson Bate. *John Keats.* Harvard University Press: Cambridge, MA, 1963, p. 49.

143   "human beings are by nature" Duncan B. Forrester, James Ian Hamilton McDonald, Gian Tellini. *Encounter with God.* T. T. Clark International: NY, 2004, p. 14.

143   "I find that I cannot" Donald C. Goellnicht. *The Poet-Physician: Keats and Medical Science.* University of Pittsburgh Press: Pittsburgh, 1984, p. 176.

144   "O, for only ten years" John Keats, "Sleep and Poetry."

145   "I would sooner fail" Jack Stillinger. *John Keats: Complete Poems.* Harvard University Press: Cambridge, 1999, p. 432.

145   "There is no greater" Peter Gordon. *The Study of Education.* Routledge: London, 1980, p. 214.

145   "A clenched fist" Keats, in Ward, *Keats,* p. 131.

145 "The high idea I have" John Keats. *Complete Works: Letters. 1901.* Nabu Press: New York, 2011, p. 38.

147 "That which is creative" Kay R. Jamison. *Touched with Fire.* Free Press: New York, 1996, p. 114.

147 "Wherein lies" John Keats, *Endymion.*

147 "A fellowship with" ibid.

148 "Several things dovetailed" Andrew Motion. *Keats.* University of Chicago Press: Chicago, 2001, p. 217.

148 "annul the self" Keats, in Ward, *Keats,* p. 161.

148 "Let us open" Keats, in Donald Goellnicht. *The Poet-Physician: Keats and Medical Science.* University of Pittsburgh Press: Pittsburgh, 1984, p. 110.

148 "A year or two earlier" Ward, *Keats,* p. 167.

148 "To bear all naked" John Keats, "Hyperion."

149 "If Poetry comes not" Bate, *Keats,* p. 234.

149 "I think a little" John Keats, Robert Gittings, Jon Mee. *John Keats: Selected Letters.* Oxford University Press: London, 2002, p. 54.

149 "not for Fame and Laurel" Gittings, *Keats,* p. 224.

149 "Being a poet" Ward, *Keats,* p. 224.

150 "We often spoke" personal letter to the author from John Stevenson.

151 "I got to see Mark" ibid.

152 "to bear all naked truths" Keats, "Hyperion."

152 "the supreme experience" Gerald B. Kauvar. *The Other Poetry of Keats.* Associated University Press: Cranbury, New Jersey, 1969, p. 115.

152 "Do you not see" Keats, in Motion, *Keats,* p. 377.

153 "For these few weeks" Ward, *Keats,* p. 279.

153 "I look upon fine" Meg Harris Williams. *Inspiration in Milton and Keats.* Palgrave MacMillan, London, 1982, p. 165.

153 "Verse that comes not" Keats, in Ward, *Keats,* p. 320.

155 "a poem should ride" Robert Frost, in Parini, *Frost,* p. 42.

155 "I know the colour" Keats, in Ward, *Keats,* p. 347.

156 "many a verse" Keats in Stuart M. Sperry. *Keats the Poet.* Princeton University Press; Princeton, NJ, 1993, p. 79.

NINE

160 "If you stay in the center" Mitchell, *Tao,* Saying 33.

165 "He made it clear" Marion Woodman. *Bone: A Journal of Wisdom, Strength and Healing.* Penguin Putnam: New York, 2000, p. 15.

166 "When [God] is moving you" ibid., p. 11.

166 "I persevered" ibid., p. xi.

166 "Destiny is recognizing" ibid., p. xvi.

166 "These are strange days" ibid., p. 5.

167 "In his eighties" Marion Woodman. *Conscious Femininity: Interviews with Marion Woodman.* Inner City Books: Toronto, 1993, p. 108.

168   "The shadow is anything" Marion Woodman. *Dreams: Language of the Soul.* Sounds True Recordings: Boulder, CO, 1991, cassette recording no. A131.

168   "The shadow may carry" Woodman, *Dreams.*

169   "Once we know what" ibid.

169   "I put rows of dreams" Marion Woodman with Jill Mellick. *Coming Home to Myself: Daily Reflections for a Woman's Body and Soul.* Conari Press: Berkeley, 1998, p. 3.

170   "What a relief" Woodman, *Conscious Femininity,* p. 51.

170   "My dark images are" Woodman, *Bone,* p. 52.

170   "I know that this death" ibid., p. 37.

170   "In our dreams we" Marion Woodman. *Rolling Away the Stone.* Sounds True Recordings: Boulder, CO, 1989.

172   "Death is inevitable" Easwaran, *Gita, 2.28,* p. 64.

172   "I decided if I" Woodman, *Bone,* p. 66.

173   "My body has always" ibid., p. 105.

173   "The invitation into" This section is paraphrased from Woodman's description of the stages of initiation in the Preface to *Coming Home,* p. 18.

173   "We usually need" Woodman, *Coming Home,* p. 18.

174   "We learn to live" Marion Woodman. *The Pregnant Virgin: A Process of Psychological Transformation.* Inner City: Toronto, 1997, p. 51.

174   "Holding an inner" Woodman, *Coming Home,* p. 188.

176   "Died into life" Woodman, *Bone,* p. xv.

177   From "Sailing to Byzantium," by William Butler Yeats, first published 1928 in *The Tower.* Used by permission.

177   "awakens to the light" Easwaran, *Gita,* 2.69, p. 68.

177   "Cancer has made me" Woodman, *Bone,* p. xvi.

177   "Through failures" ibid., p. 296.

178   "Oh, Marion" This section adapted and quoted from Woodman, *Bone,* p. 240.

TEN

180   "Are you too deeply" Brenda Wineapple. *White Heat: The Friendship of Emily Dickinson and Thomas Wentworth Higginson.* Anchor: New York, 2009, p. 4.

181   "Before my departure" Maynard Solomon. *Late Beethoven: Music, Thought, Imagination.* University of California Press: Berkeley, 2004, p. 3.

182   "Blessed is the man" A quotation from entry number "64a" from Beethoven's *Tagebuch,* translated in its entirety in Maynard Solomon. *Beethoven Essays.* Harvard University Press: Cambridge, 1998, p. 268.

183   "Beethoven turned all of his defeats" Maynard Solomon. *Beethoven.* Schirmer Trade Books: New York, 2001, p. 161.

183   "saw the little Louis" Solomon. *Beethoven.* p. 22.

183   "[The] Beethoven children" ibid., p. 24.

184 "play for mortal stakes" Robert Frost. "Two Tramps in Mud Time," from *A Further Range*. Henry Holt: New York, 1936.

185 "From my earliest childhood" Leon Plantinga. *Beethoven's Concertos*. W. W. Norton: New York, 1999, p. 322.

185 "Since I was a child" Maynard Solomon. *Late Beethoven: Music, Thought, Imagination*. University of California Press: Berkeley, 2003, p. 93.

185 "There is hardly any" Solomon, *Beethoven*, p. 53.

185 "I have not the slightest" Stephen Rumph. *Beethoven After Napoleon*. University of California Press: Berkeley, 1994, p. 97.

186 "In whatever company" Elliot Forbes, ed. *Thayer's Life of Beethoven, Vol I.*, Revised. Princeton University Press: Princeton, 1967, p. 185.

186 "bested by that young" Solomon, *Beethoven*, p. 79.

186 "[He] was short of stature" ibid., p. 105.

187 "His mouth was small" ibid.

187 "always merry, mischievous" ibid., p. 106.

187 "Live only in your art" Solomon, *Essays, Tagebuch* entry 88, p. 274.

187 "Everything that is called life" Solomon, *Essays, Tagebuch* entry 40, p. 258.

187 His daily schedule is instructive. This section is drawn largely from Solomon's descriptions of Beethoven's interesting schedule. See Solomon, *Beethoven*, pp. 107–108 for more about Beethoven's daily life.

188 "I always have a notebook" Solomon, *Beethoven*, p. 107.

189 "thematic condensation; more" ibid., p. 141.

190 ". . . my ears continue to" David Wyn-Jones. *The Life of Beethoven*. Cambridge University Press: Cambridge, UK, 1998, p. 58.

191 "It was only my art" Forbes, *Thayer*, p. 305.

192 "With joy I hasten" Michael Black. *Crossing Out the Emperor*. Chipmunka-publishing: London, 2011, p. 55.

192 "I will take Fate" J. W. N. Sullivan. *Beethoven: His Spiritual Development*. Vintage Books: New York, 1960, p. 72.

192 "he found that his genius" Sullivan, *Beethoven*, p. 73.

192 "In the middle of winter" Albert Camus. "Return to Tipasa," *The Myth of Sisyphus and Other Essays*. Random House: New York, 1961, p. 144.

193 "Never again was" Sullivan, *Beethoven*, p. 77.

193 "In the same way" ibid.

193 "I live entirely" Barry Cooper. *Beethoven*. Oxford University Press: USA, 2008, p. 117.

194 "Submission, deepest" Solomon, *Essays, Tagebuch* number 1, p. 246.

194 "Like Henry James's" Solomon, *Beethoven*, p. 161.

194 "its unique ability" ibid., p. 250.

195 "I often despair" ibid., p. 283.

195 "I learned yesterday" Edmund Morris. *Beethoven: The Universal Composer*. HarperCollins: New York, 2005, p. 179.

196 "God sees into" Solomon, *Essays*, p. 227.

196 "Perform thy duty" Solomon, *Essays, Tagebuch* number 64a, p. 269.

196 "Let not thy life" ibid., *Tagebuch* number 64b, p. 269.

197 "My motto is always" Alessandra Comini. *The Changing Image of Beethoven: A Study in Mythmaking.* Sunstone: Santa Fe, NM, 2008, p. 69.

198 "Late in the afternoon" Solomon, *Beethoven,* p. 381.

PART V: The Fourth Pillar: "Turn It Over to God"

204 "[The Self] is not born" Stoler Miller, *Gita,* 2.20, p. 32.

205 "Creatures are unmanifest" ibid., 2.28, p. 33.

207 "From broken memory" ibid., 2.63, p. 38.

207 "Our birth is but a sleep" William Wordsworth. "Ode: Intimations of Immortality," completed in 1804 and first published in *Poems, In Two Volumes.* Longman, Hurst, Reeves Publishers: London, 1807.

207 "This is the use" T. S. Eliot, "Little Gidding" III, *The Four Quartets.*

208 "Krishna, my delusion" Stoler Miller, *Gita,* 18.73, p. 153.

208 "Sometimes, because we were" Easwaran, *Gita,* 11.41, p. 155.

209 "Just as you have described" ibid., 11.3,4, p. 150.

209 "If a thousand suns" ibid., 11.13,14, p. 151.

ELEVEN

216 "To know when to act" Easwaran, *Gita,* 18.30, p. 208.

217 "I grew up like a" Catherine Clinton. *Harriet Tubman: The Road to Freedom.* Back Bay Books: New York, 2004, p. 16.

218 "I had reasoned this" Laurie Calkhoven. *Harriet Tubman: Leading the Way to Freedom.* Sterling: New York, 2008, Chapter Three, epigraph.

217 "flying over fields and towns" Clinton, *Tubman,* p. 38.

219 "MINTY, aged about" Clinton, *Tubman,* p. 34.

221 "stationmasters" See more about these roles in Clinton, *Tubman,* p. 66.

221 "I wouldn't trust" Clinton, *Tubman,* p. 84.

222 "Harriet seems to have" Ann Petry. *Harriet Tubman: Conductor on the Underground Railroad.* Amistad: New York, 1995, p. 219.

222 "I never met" James A. McGowan. *Station Master on the Underground Railroad.* MacFarland and Co.: Jefferson, North Carolina, 2004, p. 100.

222 "When danger is near" M. J. Cosson. *Harriet Tubman.* Abdo Publishing: Minneapolis, Minnesota, 2007, p. 53.

223 "When God becomes our guide" Jean-Pierre de Caussade. *Abandonment to Divine Providence.* Translated and Introduced by John Beevers. Image Books: New York, 1975, p. 83.

223 "These actions are" author's translation, *Gita,* 18.48.

223 "When we are led" de Caussade, *Abandonment,* p. 83.

225 "Now it is surely" ibid., p. 56.

225 "This work in our souls" ibid.

228 "By fulfilling the obligations" Easwaran, *Gita,* 18.47, p. 210.

231 "The old woman was" Milton G. Sennett. *Harriet Tubman: Myth, Memory and History.* Duke University Press: Durham, NC, 2007, p. 150.

231 "I was conductor of" Laurie Calkhoven. *Harriet Tubman: Leading the Way to Freedom.* Sterling Books: New York, 2008, Chapter Eight, epigraph.

231 "If you are tired" ibid., epigraph to the Introduction.

231 "The strangest thing" Clinton, *Tubman,* p. 95.

231 "Those who follow" Easwaran, *Gita,* 5.7, 8, p. 96.

231 "Each and every person" Clinton, *Tubman,* p. 221.

TWELVE

233 "Thus came into being" Ainslee Thomas Embree, Stephen Hay, William T. De Bary. *Sources of Indian Tradition: Modern India and Pakistan.* Columbia University Press: New York, 1988, p. 266.

234 "spiritual reference book" Eknath Easwaran. *Gandhi the Man.* Nilgiri Press: Novales, California, 1997, p. 8.

234 "Every moment of Gandhi's life" Louis Fischer. *Gandhi: His Life and Message for the World.* Signet Classics: New York, 2010, p. 12.

234 "haunted by the fear" Easwaran, *Gandhi,* p. 12.

234 "Nonviolence and cowardice go ill" ibid., p. 84.

235 "It is perfectly all right" The author imagines this line.

235 "The mantra becomes" M. K. Gandhi. *Self Restraint v. Self-Indulgence.* Navajivan Publishing, 1947, p. 64.

236 "Whenever the mind wanders" Easwaran, *Gita,* 6.26, p. 107.

236 "When meditation is mastered" ibid., 6.19, p. 106.

236 "Krishna, the mind is" ibid., 6.34, p. 108.

237 "Just keep practicing" ibid., 6.35, p. 108.

238 "It went straight" ibid., p. 35.

238 "What effect this reading" M. K. Gandhi. *Autobiography: The Story of My Experiments with Truth.* Dover Publications: Mineola, New York, 1983, p. 233.

238 "When doubts haunt me" Sabapathy Kulandran. *Grace in Christianity and Hinduism.* Lutterworth Press: Cambridge, England, 2004, p. 139.

239 "inner relish, distinctly" Fischer, *Gandhi,* p. 11.

239 "His feet barely touched" ibid., p. 11.

241 "I had learnt" Richard L. Johnson, ed. *Gandhi's Experiments with Truth: Essential Writings By and About Mahatma Gandhi.* Lexington Books: Lanham, Maryland, 2005, p. 8.

241 "Without realizing it" Easwaran, *Gandhi,* p. 22.

242 "My study of English law" M. K. Gandhi. *Autobiography,* p. 233.

242 "He who devotes himself" M. K. Gandhi. *Non-Violent Resistance Satyagraha.* Dover Publications: Mineola, New York, 2001, p. 48.

242 "He will take only" M. K. Gandhi, Judith Margaret Brown. *Gandhi: The Essential Writings.* Oxford University Press: London, 2008, p. 77.

244 "Hope and fear are both" Mitchell, *Tao,* Saying 13.

245 "There comes a time" K. D. Gangrade. *The Gandhian Approach to Development and Social Works.* Concept Publishing: Columbia, Missouri, 2005, p. 18.

245 "Gandhi was the most bewildering" Easwaran, *Gandhi,* p. 65.

246 "the *satyagrahi's* object" Jai Narain Sharma. *Rediscovering Gandhi, Satyagraha Vol. 3.* Concept Publishing: Columbia, Missouri, 2008, p. 91.

247 "Greater courage is required" Easwaran, *Gandhi,* p. 84.

247 "Have I that nonviolence" M. K. Gandhi, Louis Fischer. *The Essential Gandhi: An Anthology of His Writings on His Life, Work and Ideas.* Vintage: New York, 2002, p. 319.

247 "Death is the appointed end" Louis Fischer. *The Life of Mahatma Gandhi.* Harper and Row: New York, 1983, p. 81.

248 "Select your purpose" Easwaran, *Gandhi,* p. 49.

248 "Do not resort to" ibid.

249 "Abandon all supports" Easwaran, *Gita,* 18.66, p. 212.

249 "Cast off your dependency" Eknath Easwaran, *The Bhagavad Gita.* Nilgiri Press: Novales, CA, 2009, Kindle edition, Note #41, p. 275.

Epilogue

250 "Have you understood" Easwaran, *Gita,* 18.72, p. 212.

251 "You have dispelled" ibid., 18.73, p. 212.

251 "Free from self-will" ibid., 18.53-56, pp. 210-211.

254 "We cannot master" Thomas Merton. *No Man is an Island.* Harcourt, Brace: New York, 1978, p. 130.

254 ". . . the fulfillment of every" ibid., p. 137.

255 ". . . we cannot achieve greatness" ibid., p. 122.

255 "Whenever I remember" Easwaran, *Gita,* 18.76–77, p. 213.

256 "Wherever the divine Krishna" ibid., 18.78, p. 213.

ABOUT THE TYPE

This book was set in Minion, a 1990 Adobe Originals typeface by Robert Slimbach. Minion is inspired by classical, old style typefaces of the late Renaissance, a period of elegant, beautiful, and highly readable type designs. Created primarily for text setting, Minion combines the aesthetic and functional qualities that make text type highly readable with the versatility of digital technology.